Springer-Verlag Wien GmbH

Acta Neurochirurgica
Supplements

Editor: H.-J. Steiger

Joint Residency Advisory and Accreditation Commitee (JRAAC)
A Joint Commitee of the the U.E.M.S. and E.A.N.S.

Training in Neurosurgery in the Countries of the EU

A Guide to Organize a Training Programme

Edited by
H.-J. Reulen

in collaboration with
J. Brennum, Fl. Gjerris, J. Haase, W. Kanpolat, D. Lang, K. W. Lindsay,
J. Lobo Antunes, D. W. Long, G. Neil Dwyer, G. Schackert,
J. Steers, H.-J. Steiger, J. C. Tonn, T. Trojanowski, and P. A. Winkler

Acta Neurochirurgica
Supplement 90

Springer-Verlag Wien GmbH

Univ.-Prof. Dr. H.-J. Reulen
Neurochirurgische Uni.-Klinik, Klinikum Großhadern, Munich, Germany

Originally published by SpringerWienNewYork 2004
Softcover reprint of the hardcover 1st edition 2004

Typesetting: Asco Typesetters, Hong Kong

Printed on acid-free and chlorine-free bleached paper

SPIN: 10992920

Library of Congress Control Number: 2004109046

With 4 Figures

ISBN 978-3-7091-7214-8 ISBN 978-3-7091-0633-4 (eBook)
DOI 10.1007/978-3-7091-0633-4

Preface

The idea for this book was born during the discussions of JRAAC following certification visits to a number of different neurosurgical departments all over Europe. The members of JRAAC realized recurrent problems in the structure of training programmes on the one side an many positive solutions on the other side. The idea evolved to compile a manual or practical guide, respectively, how to solve such typical problems. Hence this book is a common effort of the members of JRAAC to provide advice and support to those involved in the organisation of neurosurgical education.

The new Neurosurgical Training Charter of the UEMS, as presented in Chapter II, defines now a "European Model" to *structure* a training programme with a clear set of standards and requirements. This is inevitably necessary if we want to move toward a steady improvement of neurosurgical education in Europe. It should be emphasized that this concerns the *external* structure, the skeleton. The *internal* structure of a programme, the curriculum, the content of the various training years, the philosophy of a department, the formation of an educational environment, etc. remain still in the responsibility of the department. Both together determine the charm and attractiveness of a department.

The chapters in this volume cover most of the mentioned "standards and requirements" asked for in the new UEMS Training Charter. The solutions offered are based on many years of personal experience of the authors as well as good examples encountered over the years in the different departments. The book may be used as a guide by those departments that are in the process of developing or improving their training programme. But also departments with an already advanced programme will find a variety of important information. The solutions offered may be used as they are or be modified and adjusted to the local situation.

We wish good luck and success in your endeavours.

For the members of JRAAC

H.-J. Reulen

Contents

Listed in Current Contents

Acta Neurochir (2004) [Suppl] 90: 1–2

Printed in Austria

Introduction

J. Lobo Antunes

Serviço de Neurocirurgia, Hospital de Santa Maria, Lisboa, Portugal

One of the main concerns of the founding fathers of the European Association of Neurosurgical Societies (EANS) was certainly to contribute to improving toward the quality of neurosurgical education in Europe. We were then living in a politically divided continent with striking asymmetries in the quality of care delivered to the various populations.

Today we are experiencing the dawn of a new period, not only because the European Union will soon encompass twenty five countries, but because we have witnessed the progressive disappearance of the political, economical, and educational barriers and a totally new mobility of students and professionals, although it is true that from its inception, EANS knew no frontiers. But at the same time we recognize the need to face the new challenges that the increasing sophistication of training in our speciality definitely pose.

Some of us, who for many years have been members of the juries of the European Examinations, have recognized that there still remains remarkable disparity in the quality of training in the various countries, which is certainly, at least in part, due to different educational methodologies and a rather incipient concern about the need to assess what is being accomplished. We are fully aware that it is crucial for each country to preserve its own culture and tradition, and that neurosurgeons carry on their work in a specific social, economic, and professional context. But in a Europe without frontiers, it is important to define a set of requirements of training and professional experience that may allow us to define a "European model", which inevitably will have to be drawn by the wise contribution of all countries involved.

Hans-Jürgen Reulen who was, until recently, the Chairman of the Joint Residency and Advisory and Accrediation Committee had the foresight to recognise these new paths in neurosurgical education and the need to join efforts with the Union Européenne des Médecins Specialistes and set up the criteria that would allow the recognition of excellence of the various European services, by a demanding and rigorous process of certification.

The present guide is the logical development of that effort and will be most helpful to any person involved in the education and training of young neurosurgeons. It is devoid of the usual verbiage of educational handbooks: it is a practical guidebook addressing the needs of anybody in charge of this wonderful, almost magic, task of making a neurosurgeon with enough cognitive information and technical skills but also with all the other ingredients that define us as a unique brand of doctors including what is part of the so-called "hidden curriculum".

This publication is particularly interesting also because it collects the experiences of people who have been working in these areas for many years and have different backgrounds and cultural heritages. But this is the fascination of our old continent!

As I mentioned, the basic goal of this publication was to make it a practical guide, so naturally some topics which are complementary to the education of a young neurosurgeon, such as uncertainty and error, risk management or dealing with conflicts of interest, were deliberately left out. But it will give the reader the basic tools to structure a neurosurgical service, following simple principles and a common language which will help to achieve one of the aspiring goals of the EANS: excellence in what we do.

I further believe we are anticipating what will soon become a political mandate – to harmonize specialty training in Europe, to allow the development of uniform criteria for a European accreditation, and guarantee the free circulation of skilled professionals. And this was what our founding fathers envisioned many years ago.

J. Lobo Antunes
Past President of the EANS

Acta Neurochir (2004) [Suppl] 90: 3–11

Printed in Austria

I UEMS charter on training of medical specialists in the EU – the new neurosurgical training charter

J. Steers[1], **H.-J. Reulen**[2], and **K. W. Lindsay**[3]

[1] Department of Clinical Neurosciences, Western General Hospital, Edingburgh, UK
[2] Department of Neurosurgery, Klinikum Großhadern, Ludwig-Maximilians-University, Munich, Germany
[3] Department of Neurosurgery, Southern General Hospital, Glasgow, UK

In the Directive 93/16 EEC of 5.04.1993, the European Commission laid down the general guidelines for the training of medical specialists in the member states of the EU, EFTA and associated member states. On the European level, the UEMS (European Union of Medical Specialists) is responsible for harmonisation and improvement of the quality of medical specialist practice in the EU. Its statutory purpose is the formulation of a common policy in the field of training.

In 1995 the "Charter on Training of Medical Specialists in the European Community" was published, outlining the general requirements and guidelines of postgraduate training as well as the special requirements for the various medical specialities including neurosurgery (www.uems.be → Training/Formation). Responsible national organisations have strongly been recommended to implement these requirements and guidelines in their national training programmes.

On request of the UEMS, a novellation was formulated in 2002–2004 for all medical specialities which is now available also for the field of neurosurgery. It describes more precisely then so far the structures of neurosurgical training including the external audits required now. The present version at the time of publication of this book has not definitely been ratified yet so that minor alterations are still possible. Also, the operative figures required at the end of training have not yet been finalised. Therefore the chapter does not contain the appendix 1+2, mentioned on page 11/12. However, we thought it necessary to include the new *Neurosurgical Training Charter* since it will be the working basis for the JRAAC and above all for the national societies and national authorities.

This document will be the professional position paper needed by the European Commission when further EU directives in the field of medical specialist practice are being contemplated.

Correspondence: J. Steers, Department of Clinical Neurosciences, Western General Hospital, Crewe Road, Edingburgh, EH4 2SU, UK. e-mail: js@skull.dcn.ed.ac.uk

Charter on training of medical specialists in the EU – Requirements for the speciality of neurosurgery (as of February 28th, 2004). (UEMS Specialist Section of Neurosurgery)

Foreword

This document sets out standards and guidelines for neurosurgical residency training and for approval of training programmes in the countries of the EU/EFTA and associated member states. It is recognised that there are a number of structural and operational differences in the health care systems, appointment procedures and training systems in these different countries. This document provides the basis for the development of a harmonised, comprehensive, structured and balanced training programme in Neurosurgery.

The future of European neurosurgery will depend on the quality of training offered to our trainees. Apprentice style training, which has been at the heart of traditional training, is increasingly being threatened by regulation and legislation. Hours of work for both trainers and trainees is coming under increasing pressure from many competing demands, many of which further fragment the training opportunities available.

It is recognized that in future there may be a need to prolong the training time in clinical neurosurgery from 4 to 5 years.

Goal of training programme

The primary goal of a training programme is to provide the trainee with a broad knowledge base, the necessary operative and procedural skills and experience as well as professional judgement for independent neurosurgical practice; a further goal is to teach him/her self-criticism, critical assessment of his/her results, the ability to self-directed learning which will eventually lead to continued growth, expert practice and professionalism.

Definition of speciality

Neurosurgery is a discipline that provides the diagnosis, the operative, and non-operative management (i.e. prevention, diagnosis, evaluation, treatment, intensive care, and rehabilitation) of patients with pathological processes that affect the central, peripheral (and autonomic) nervous system, including their supporting structures and vascular supply as well as the operative and non-operative management of pain. This encompasses the modern treatment of disorders of the brain, meninges, skull and their blood supply including the extracranial carotid and vertebral arteries; disorders of the pituitary gland, disorders of the cranial, spinal nerves, peripheral nerves and disorders of the autonomic nervous system, disorders of the spinal cord, meninges and spine including those which may require treatment by spinal fusion or instrumentation.

Article 1: General rules on monitoring and accreditation

1.1 Manpower planning

Manpower planning should be developed, based on the demands and provision of safe neurosurgical care across the countries of the EU and associated member states. Planners will have to take into consideration demographic changes in any given population such as its growth and ageing, changing treatment modalities and actual workload, the possible effects of legislation on working hours and, in some centers, the involvement in education of medical professionals. Whilst many countries intend to increase the number of trained neurosurgeons, there is a recognised risk that overproduction leads to the dilution of experience and consequent difficulties in maintaining competencies.

1.2 Monitoring authority at European level

Harmonisation of neurosurgical training throughout Europe will require standards of training and monitoring, and centralised registration of approval of neurosurgical training programmes in the EU and associated countries. The central monitoring body is the **J**oint **R**esidency **A**dvisory and **A**ccreditation **C**ommittee (JRAAC); a joint committee of the Section of Neurosurgery of the UEMS and the European Association of Neurosurgical Societies (EANS).

National professional bodies (responsible for the recognition of medical specialists in individual countries) can monitor and recognise neurosurgical training programmes using UEMS standards based on the training charter. In the interest of developing common standards, cooperation with JRAAC is recommended.

1.3 Accreditation of training institutions

The visiting and evaluation of training institutions is an important feed back mechanism for quality improvement.

1.3.1 A training institution or training programme must have European or national recognition/ accreditation, respectively, according to UEMS/ national standards.

1.3.2 To be accredited, an educational programme must substantially comply with the special requirements for residency training in neurosurgery as set down by the UEMS Training Charter.

Programmes must demonstrate their compliance with these requirements at the time of the site visit. Site visits will be carried out in accordance with the Charter on Site Visits.

1.3.4 Nationally accredited training programmes in neurosurgery may also be approved by the Joint Residency Advisory and Accreditation Committee.

1.3.5 A training programme must be reviewed every 5 years, or within 12 months following the appointment of a new director of training programme.

1.4 Accreditation of trainers

Trainers must be certified neurosurgeons and the Programme Director must be registered in accordance with the medical licensing authority of the country of the training programme and possess the necessary administrative, teaching and clinical skills required to conduct the programme.

Article 2: General aspects of training in the speciality

2.1 Selection for and access to the speciality

2.1.1 Applicants should have a valid license to practice medicine within a training programme in EU and associated countries; this license has to be recognised by the country where he/she will be trained.

Training institutions or, if present, responsible bodies should select or appoint trainees suitable for the speciality in accordance with an established selection procedure. This selection procedure should be transparent and fair, and application should be open to all eligible persons. The candidates should be aware of these requirements.

2.1.2 After appointment of a trainee, a training agreement should be entered into by the Director of the Programme and trainee and duly signed by the trainee and the Director. The agreement should define – in terms of education and training – the relationships, duties and obligations on each side.

2.2 Duration of training

Training must cover the full range of the speciality and lead to the ability for independent practice on completion of training.

2.2.1 Neurosurgical training is of 6 years minimum duration and consists of a minimum of 4 years' training in clinical neurosurgery in an accredited programme. Of these 4 years dedicated to neurosurgery, at least 3 years should be spent in a UEMS member state and not less than 3 years in the same recognised programme. Training must include adequate exposure to intensive care and to pediatric neurosurgery (see 3.2.1).

2.2.2 Up to a total of two years may be spent in related disciplines (in a surgical discipline, in neurology, in neuropediatrics, in neuroradiology, in neuropathology, in neurophysiology) and/or activities including research in neurosciences.

2.3 Curriculum of general and specific training periods

2.3.1 A written *Training Curriculum* must be designed to provide a diversified and balanced quality (theoretical and practical) of neurosurgical education describing the contents and aims in each year of training. This must be available to trainees and the faculty. Emphasis should be placed on adequate time allocated for study and tuition independent of clinical duties. It may be necessary for some units to formally organize specific training periods in associated neurosurgical units, if adequate experience cannot be provided internally.

2.3.2 There should be established *Rotation Periods* covering all main areas of neurosurgery (including pediatric neurosurgery). These rotations should be organized in such a way as to give trainees increasing responsibility as they progress through their training with regard to patient care and surgical experience. Rotations may include neurology, surgical disciplines, neuroradiology, neuropathology, radiosurgery, etc., neurosciences or research, depending on requirements, local availability and the department's emphasis.

2.3.3 Some institutions may wish to use a structured *Surgical Training Plan*. The main idea of this is a continuous and systemic escalation of surgical responsibilities and competence through training years 1–6.

2.3.4 Education programme

There should be a documented, continuous *Education Programme* throughout the training, which should include daily, weekly and monthly conferences, etc. There must be protected time for study and tuition.

This Education Programme should consist of

- A programme of lectures including visiting speakers
- Clinical presentations from all neuroscience disciplines
- Neuropathological and neuroradiological conferences
- Journal club
- Mortality and morbidity conference (with audited attendance)
- Research meetings
- Regular teaching conferences including subspecialities (residents should take increasing responsibility in the conferences and in the teaching of junior trainees, nurses, students)
- Teaching in ethics, administration, management and economics

2.3.5 Exposure to research

Trainees should be encouraged to undertake research and would be expected to develop an understanding of research methodology. An appropriately qualified person should supervise specific research projects. There should be a protected period of time within a 6-year-programme where a trainee can participate in a specific research project. All trainees will be expected to be able to assess published work. In academic programmes, clinical and/or basic research opportunities must be available to the trainee with appropriate faculty supervision.

2.3.6 Participation in meetings/courses

It is recommended that trainees attend the meetings of the national neurosurgical society once a year (or an equivalent meeting). If possible trainees should participate in the European Association of Neurosurgical Societies' training courses or equivalent national training courses. During their training, they should also attend a subspecialty course/meeting (spinal, stereotaxy, paediatric, peripheral nerves, neurooncology, neurovascular, etc.) and if possible a hands-on-course in anatomy or surgical techniques.

2.3.7 Trainees should keep a *Trainee Portfolio* containing details of previous training posts, examinations passed, lists of publications and presentations at meetings, courses attended, cumulative operative totals, copies of assessment forms of these different training periods.

2.4 Training log-book and periodic progress assessment of trainees

2.4.1 Log-Book

Each trainee must keep an authorised *Log-Book* that meets the standards of the EANS/UEMS logbook for documentation of operative experience. The trainee will have to demonstrate that he/she has assisted a wide range of cases which should include a balance of trainer assisted and personal cases under supervision. Log-book entries must be monitored by regular inspection and signed off by the appropriate trainer. The log-book must be available at Board examination.

2.4.2 Periodic progress assessment

The purpose of assessment is to ensure continuing progress in the trainee's knowledge and skills as well as professional conduct and ethics.

Trainees have to meet the agreed standards and requirements of the planned programme. Assessment must be performed on a six monthly basis or at the end of each rotation period by the appropriate trainer in writing using an evaluation sheet. The log-book is used as supporting documentation. The result of the evaluation must be discussed with each resident. Failure to meet agreed targets must be brought to the attention of the training programme director.

It is the responsibility of the training programme director to identify any failure in a trainee's progress, to conduct and to provide appropriate advice, and to take remedial action.

In the event of trainees not progressing as required, there are three stages of remedial action. Targeted training: closer monitoring and supervision to address particular needs; intensified supervision and, if necessary, repetition of the appropriate part of the programme; and finally the potential to withdraw a trainee from the programme.

It is of the greatest importance that accurate records of the trainees' progress are kept (trainee's portfolio).

In future a parallel assessment for trainees to assess their training may be introduced to monitor the effectiveness of the training programme.

Article 3: Requirements for training institutions

3.1 Process for recognition as a training institution

In order to be recognised, the training institution must substantially comply with the special requirements for Residency Training in Neurosurgery and the General Requirements in Graduate Medical Education of the UEMS Training Charter. The training institution (programme) must be able to demonstrate its compliance with these requirements at the time of a site visit conducted by the JRAAC or equivalent national body.

3.1.1 The application

The Programme Director must submit a Programme Application Form to JRAAC describing the personnel, space, technical facilities, and in particular the Residency Training Programme. The Application Form can be obtained from the secretary of JRAAC or the web site of EANS (www.eans.org → What's new → Accreditation of Training Centers).

3.1.2 The site visit

The next step will be a site visit of the applicant institution, conducted by two independent visitors nominated by JRAAC and a third national observer/visitor appointed by the applicant institution. The date of the site visit will be arranged between the Programme Director and the site visitors. The Programme Director will receive the necessary information to prepare the site visit in due time. The site visit will be performed in accordance with the guidelines of the UEMS Charter on Visitation of Training Centers.

The site visit serves to explore in detail the training programme, the educational and scientific environment, by holding discussions with the Chairman, the teachers, the trainees, and administration of the unit. A report will be prepared by the site visitors and will be part of the final decision of the unit on the accreditation status of the programme. All information obtained during the interviews with trainers and trainees remains absolutely confidential.

The accreditation status as decided by the JRAAC will be reported to the Programme Director by formal Letter of Notification. Together with the site visit report, additional advice and recommendations – if necessary – will be given to further improve the Training Programme.

3.1.3 The accreditation

The following decisions may be taken by the JRAAC with regard to the accreditation status of a Training Institution and Programme:

Full accreditation may be granted if the programme has demonstrated its full compliance with the European Training Charter. The Department will receive a certificate indicating that the Department and the Training Programme fulfill the criteria meeting European Standards of Excellence for Education in Neurosurgery. The accreditation shall be re-assessed after 5 years or within one year after change of Programme Director.

Provisional accreditation indicates that the programme is basically in line (but not in compliance) with the requirements and standards. It is considered to be at the development stage of its training programme. The Programme Director will be requested to submit a so-called Progress Report within one or two years of notification. The Committee shall specify precisely the information to be provided. When a Progress Report is requested, a specific due date should be included in the request.

Accreditation may be withheld if the programme does not substantially comply with the requirements and standards. The Committee will cite those areas in which the reviewed programme does not comply with the standards. A new application can be submitted when the areas indicated are brought into compliance with the requirements and standards.

Accreditation may be discontinued if a programme for some reason is no longer in compliance with the requirements and standards. A new application can be submitted if the requirements are again fulfilled.

Reassessment of a Programme is usually done after 5 years or within one year after a change of Programme Director.

3.2 Requirements on equipment and educational facilities

3.2.1 The training programme

- There must be a referral base sufficient to provide an adequate case volume and mixture to support the training programme.
- There must be a minimum of 4 trainers (including chairman/programme director).
- There must be at least 30 neurosurgical beds, and in addition critical care beds (7–10 per million).
- There must be at least two designated fully staffed (neurosurgically trained staff) and appropriately equipped operating theatres with availability of a 24 hour operating theatre.
- There must be an operating microscope with CCTV for each theatre. The following are deemed to be essential equipment: ultrasonic aspirator, image guidance, a stereotactic system, radiological imaging, endoscopy equipment, ultrasound equipment as standard. Laser equipment may be necessary for specialised procedures.
- Neurosurgical theatres should be covered by anaesthetists with a special interest in neuroanaesthesia. Anaesthesia cover should be available at all times for neurosurgery.
- There must be designated and fully staffed neurosurgical intensive care beds. Neurosurgical intensive care may be managed by neurosurgery or there may be joint responsibility between neurosurgery and anaesthesia.
- There must be an emergency unit with 24 hrs admission.
- There must be outpatient clinics where non-emergency patients are seen before and after surgical procedures.
- There must be exposure to paediatric neurosurgery as a mandatory component of a training programme. Where this does not form part of routine work of the neurosurgical department, a six-month-secondment to an appropriate paediatric programme should be arranged.
  It must be recognised that in some European states paediatrics requires special training and a protected environment.
- There should be opportunity to obtain experience of functional neurosurgery either within the department or in another neurosurgical department specialised in this field.

Highly specialised centres not covering the whole neurosurgical field can be included in rotational systems but cannot be training centres in their own right.

3.2.2 Associations and access to other relevant specialities

Allied specialities must be present to a sufficient extent to provide the trainee with the opportunity of developing his/her skills in a team approach to patient care. The training programme should be closely associated with the following departments or units officially certified for training:

a department of neurology
a department of surgery and traumatology to support neurosurgical involvement in cranial and spinal trauma
a department of anaesthesiology with special responsibility for neuroanaesthesiology
a department of radiology
a department or unit of neuroradiology which has: imaging techniques with dedicated CT-scanning, access to MR-scanning on site and appropriate angiography equipment for diagnostic procedures including availability of interventional radiology
a department of pathology
a department or unit of neuropathology
a department of radiotherapy
a department of internal medicine and/or oncology
a department of paediatrics

3.2.3 Educational facilities

Easily accessible library with an adequate selection of books and journals on neurosurgery (mandatory)
Office space for both faculty and trainees
Facilities for computer literature searches
Space and opportunity for practical and theoretical study (mandatory)
Space and equipment for practical training of techniques in a laboratory setting
Space, equipment and supporting personnel for clinical and/or basic research in academic programmes.

3.3 Institutional quality management provisions

A training institution must have an internal system of medical audit or quality assurance.

3.3.1 Internal regulations. There should be written general guidelines of the training institution concerning patient care and patient information (patient's consent), referrals, medical records, documentation, on-call and back-up schedules, days off, residents' work schedules, attendance at conferences and educational activities. These should be available to staff and trainees.

3.3.2 Internal medical quality assurance. There must be an internal system of medical audit, such as mortality and morbidity conferences, together with a structured procedure for reporting of accidents.

3.3.3 The hospital should have measures in place (perhaps in the form of a committee) in relation to quality control such as infection control and drugs and therapeutics committee should exist.

3.3.4 A programme and training in risk management should be in place.

3.3.5 The hospital or the training institution should have an annual activities report.

Article 4: Requirements for training programme director and trainers

4.1 Criteria for training programme director

4.1.1 A Training Programme requires the appointment of a Training Programme Director to coordinate the training activities of the unit.

4.1.2 The Training Programme Director does not need to be the head of the training institution.

4.1.3 He/she must be a certified specialist of a minimum of 5 years. His/her substantial working contract must be with the training institution.

4.1.4 The CV of the Programme Director should provide evidence of continuing professional development (CPD).

4.1.5 The Programme Director must have full secretarial and administrative support and there must be sufficient protected time to carry out his/her responsibilities.

4.2 Responsibilities of training programme director

He has to

4.2.1 establish a transparent and fair selection and appointment process for trainees.

4.2.2 arrange a balanced training programme with established rotations ensuring that the trainee will have complete exposure to all aspects of neurosurgery. The programme must be written and available to trainers and trainees.

4.2.3 ensure that there is dedicated time allocated to the trainers for training and that the trainers are fulfilling their training responsibilities.

4.2.4 oversee the process of periodic assessment and review of the trainees.

4.2.5 ensure that the individual trainees' documentation (training portfolios) are up to date.

4.2.6 ensure that trainees attend appropriate and approved courses.

4.2.7 provide valid documentation as to the satisfactory completion of training.

4.2.8 ensure the annual collection and compilation of the number and types of neurosurgical operative procedures performed in the department and also in participating units connected with the training programme.

4.2.9 provide opportunity for research, audit and other educationally valid activities such as opportunities to attend training courses and scientific meetings.

4.3 Criteria for neurosurgical trainers

4.3.1 Trainers should be certified neurosurgeons who can demonstrate that they are in compliance with the requirements of continuing professional development.

4.3.2 Trainers should possess the necessary administrative, teaching and clinical skills, and commitment to conduct the programme.

4.3.3 Trainers should have undertaken instruction in training (learning needs and teaching objectives) and assessment of trainees.

4.3.4 Trainers should provide evidence of scholarly activities (clinical and/or basic research, publications in recognised journals and participation in neurosurgical scientific meetings).

4.3.5 Trainers will require secretarial and administrative support.

4.4 Responsibilities of neurosurgical trainers

They have to

4.4.1 set realistic aims and objectives for a rotation or training period

4.4.2 supervise the day to day work of the trainee on the ward, in clinic and in the operating theatre

4.4.3 support and assess trainees' surgical progress and supervise trainees' log-books

4.4.4 assess and report on trainees' progress at the end of each rotation or training period

4.4.5 ensure that the assessments and reports are documented and signed both by the trainer and the trainee

4.4.6 inform the programme director of problems at an early stage.

Article 5: Requirements for trainees

5.1 Minimal/optimal numbers

Trainees during their training must be exposed to at least 4 different trainers and the full spectrum of neurosurgical procedures.

Appendix 1 lists the minimal and optimal numbers of procedures that trainees should have performed at completion of training.

Trainees should have been directly involved in the pre- and post-operative management of these patients and should have a detailed understanding of the pre-operative investigation.

Many of the above procedures demand the use of the operating microscope with which the trainee must be fully familiar.

In addition to the above list of operative procedures, the trainees should have assisted in or partly performed operations for:

- pituitary microadenomas
- complex basal meningiomas
- arterio-venous malformations
- paediatric procedures – supra and infra-tentorial tumours
- spinal conditions

5.2 Communication abilities

- the trainee must demonstrate ability to record and convey patient details of history, examination and investigative findings to senior staff
- consent patients for operative procedures listed in 5.1 clearly detailing the reasons for performing the procedure and the risks involved
- communicate with patients and relatives and of passing on distressing information (e.g. malignancy or bereavement) in a sensitive and caring manner.

5.3 Log-book and assessment

5.3.1 The trainee must maintain an operative log book detailing his/her involvement in all cases.

5.3.2 The trainee should keep a training portfolio, which should include an up-to-date curriculum vitae incorporating

- details of previous training posts, dates, duration and trainers
- details of examinations passed
- list of publications with copies of published first page (abstract)
- list of research presentations at local, national and international meetings
- list of courses attended
- cumulative operative totals
- copies of assessment forms for each training period, completed and signed by trainers for that period

5.4 Specifications of training

The formal basis is the Training Curriculum of the department with training periods covering all main areas of neurosurgery. During his/her training, a trainee may wish to emphasise academic or research exposure or a particular area of subspecialisation. This can be organised with the Programme Director if the trainee's progress and performance allows for this, and the rotation may be adapted correspondingly. In future more trainees may wish to acquire higher competence in a subspeciality area after finishing their formal 6-year-training. This may be organised through so-called fellowship programmes.

5.5 Certifications for individual techniques/ procedures

The training record (Appendix 2) lists procedures required for neurosurgical training and indicates the minimal competency required at the end of six years' training. On completion of training, the trainee must tabulate his/her cumulative operative totals and indicate his/her level of competence. The training programme may require completion of this form at the end of each year of training.

At the end of neurosurgical training, the Training Director will certify as to the attainment of:

- satisfactory operative totals (in conjunction with Appendix 1)
- adequate competency level for each procedure (Appendix 2)
- satisfactory assessment forms for each year of training

Appendix 1 and 2 are not yet finalised.

Article 6: Certification of completion of training

The National Authority is the responsible body for recognition/certification of medical specialities in each member state of the EC/EFTA. Several of these countries now have a compulsory Board Examination. This is usually an oral examination, which is one method of assessing knowledge, clinical judgement and the candidates' thought processes. This is however not a standardized test. An examination at the end of training will become compulsory in the near future due to EU legislation. National bodies should therefore note the existence of the EANS 2-part examination (written and oral) with sessions twice a year, which leads to European certification. This may be a useful tool which could be assimilated by countries which do not have board certification examination arrangements in place, although at the time of writing, European certification is not recognised as being equivalent to national certification.

Subspecialisation

Training is a continuing process. Competence in complex procedures exceeding the operative totals and competence levels of appendices 1 and 2 can be developed either during the subspecialisation year or more likely after completion of training within the frame of a $1 - 1\frac{1}{2}$ year subspecialisation fellowship.

Correspondence: Prof. Dr. H.-J. Reulen, Schwojer Str. 19, 81249 München, Germany. e-mail: Ilona.Anders@med.uni-muenchen.de

Acta Neurochir (2004) [Suppl] 90: 13–16

Printed in Austria

II Neurosurgical training programme director position and responsibilities

G. Neil-Dwyer[1], D. A Lang[1], and T. Trojanowski[2]

[1] Wessex Neurological Centre, Southampton, UK
[2] Department of Neurosurgery, University Medical School, Lublin, Poland

In considering this key post in a training programme a few introductory remarks need to be made. The training programme needs to have an aim and a direction so that it can produce a well qualified, well trained and accredited Neurosurgeon capable of working in a multi professional environment. The training programme needs to be structured with progress monitored against clear objectives with trainees aware of their career pathways and goals. The training programme should be fair, flexible, transparent and there should be quality assurance of the programme. To achieve such a training programme requires commitment, vision and above all patience.

The appointment of a programme director for neurosurgical training

A Training Programme Director needs to be appointed to each neurosurgical training scheme. In many European countries the appointment as Programme Director is made by National Medical Authorities responsible for postgraduate education while in some it is made by the Dean of the University or the Postgraduate Dean who is responsible for postgraduate education. In many countries the Chairman automatically is considered to be the Programme Director. However, this linkage is not necessary and the appointment may take place with a nomination from the certified trainers who take part in the training programme. The appointment will normally be for a period of five years with possible re-election.

The criteria for a neurosurgical programme director

It is important to recognise that the Director of Training need not be the Head of the Department. In fact in many ways it is advisable to separate the two functions because their commitments are different and having one individual to perform both tasks will inevitably produce areas of conflict. The proposed Director should be a certified specialist for a minimum of five years, should have worked full-time within the department (s) central to the training programme. The CV of the proposed Director should provide evidence of current and continuing scientific work with some indication as to his/her commitment to training.

Importantly an Assistant Training Director must be appointed and should be a certified specialist for a minimum of five years.

The Director must have full secretarial and administrative support for this task and it should be quite separate from his/her clinical commitment. It is vital that designated time be allocated to ensure that Programme Directors have sufficient protected time to carry out their responsibilities.

The responsibilities of a training programme director

One of the principal responsibilities of the Programme Director will be to establish a transparent and fair selection and appointment process for trainees. In setting up this process the Director needs to have a clear idea of the profile of the type of candidate suitable for the training programme and in coming to this conclusion he/she will need to have discussed this with the other trainers. The Director will have to decide on basic qualifications, the mandatory educational, personal and character requirements as well as important and contributory requirements which may be helpful in a trainee if the aims of the training programme are to be achieved. It is also important that those applying for the training post are aware of the requirements.

It is the inherent responsibility of the Director to arrange and have written a carefully considered and balanced training programme which addresses the changing and progressive educational and training needs of each trainee throughout their training period.

The Director will need to organise an academic programme (lectures, research meetings, demonstrations, audit reviews, mortality and morbidity meetings) which is a central part of the trainee's educational programme. Trainees should be encouraged to be involved in the organisation of these academic sessions.

A period of time in research may benefit the trainee. In deciding on whether this should be part of an individual trainee's programme a Director will need to be certain of a number of factors. These are the trainee's ability not only academically but also in terms of being able to complete a project in time. The Director needs to know that the project is well designed, will be supervised effectively, has clearly defined and timed end-points and is properly funded. It goes without saying that the trainee will need to be enthusiastic.

After the appointment of a trainee a training agreement must be completed by the Director and signed by the trainee and the Director. This is an educational contract and should provide the trainee with an overview of his/her training.

The responsibilities of a programme directors to trainees

Their main responsibility must be to organise and co-ordinate the training programme. The trainees must be aware of all the processes and requirements of their training. The organisation and progression throughout training will need to recognise the needs of the trainee and a degree of flexibility will be required. Directors will need to provide leadership and assist in the assessment of trainees on a six monthly basis. In achieving this they will need to organise the trainees' appraisal processes, assess the competence of trainees and ensure that all trainees training portfolios are up to date. This will include signed reports, evaluation records and completed and signed logbooks. There is a European Evaluation Sheet and a logbook developed by the Joint Residency Advisory and Accreditation Committee (JRAAC) – a Joint Committee of the UEMS and EANS. The trainee will need to provide valid documentary evidence of the satisfactory completion of training. Throughout all this process the Programme Director needs to monitor, counsel and inform both the trainees and trainers.

It would be advisable, as a means of enhancing the evaluation of the effectiveness of the training programme, to have a parallel assessment form for trainees to assess their training. This assessment should be monitored by both the Director and the Authority responsible for the recognition of the programme.

The promotion of an ethos of a high level of professional conduct and ethics is mandatory within the training programme and although this lies within the remit of the Director, it must be a shared responsibility between the Director, the Trainers and the Trainees.

The responsibilities of a programme director to trainers

The Programme Director will need to ensure that all trainers have the appropriate training and support. If necessary they should arrange for trainers to attend "Training the Trainers" courses and other educational courses considered to be relevant. The Director has to ensure that trainers are fulfilling their training obligations, and, importantly, make certain that relevant documentation (assessments, logbooks) is completed in a timely (contemporaneous) fashion. The Director will also need to evaluate the effectiveness of education provision and ensure that the necessary resource elements are in place.

The responsibilities of a programme director to the training board

The Training Programme Director will need to make certain that the training programme's functions are agreed and to inform the Authority responsible for the recognition of the programme (JRAAC, National Board).

In this respect the Director will need to ensure that each training post delivers the education and training expected and agreed for that period.

The Director needs to advise the local administration or authorities on the facilities required for training and to point out any deficiency that will effect their ability to deliver the training programme.

There is also the major responsibility of organising and preparing the Unit for site inspections by authorised visitors. The Director will have the onerous task of identifying and reporting failing trainees and trainers to the responsible Training Board. The Director will be aware that for trainees who are not progressing there are recognised remedial options. These are targeted training, closer monitoring and supervision to address particular needs, intensified supervision and, if necessary, a repeat of the appropriate part of the programme and finally withdrawal from the programme. It will need to be established that any failing trainee or trainer has been made aware of the reasons for their failure, there should be evidence to demonstrate that attempts have been made to correct the problems, bearing in mind the possible remedial options, and in spite of these efforts the situation has not changed. Under these circumstances the Director has no alternative but to take the matter to the Dean and/or the responsible Training Authority.

The criteria for neurosurgical trainers

The Programme Director will need to develop with the help of colleagues and the Dean the criteria for neurosurgical trainers. A trainer should be a certified specialist, be committed to and familiar with the requirement of the training programme. The Director needs to ensure that trainers recognise their responsibilities and can reconcile them with service pressures. Directors should also recognise that trainers will require secretarial and administrative support to carry out the tasks and they should ensure that the necessary resources are made available.

The responsibilities of neurosurgical trainers

The responsibilities of the trainer should be very clearly laid out and the training programme should be available to the trainee.

It is essential that a trainer meets at an early stage their trainee and establishes their experience and identifies their learning needs. The trainer and the trainee should set realistic aims and objectives for the next six months or rotation. These should be documented and signed by both the trainer and trainee. The trainer needs to have the time to supervise the day to day work of the trainee on the ward, in the clinic and in the operating theatre. It needs to be recognised that training trainees takes up time and this must be taken into consideration in balancing the service requirements. The trainer will assess the trainee's surgical competency and knowledge on a continual basis and at the end of the six month training period or rotation, either by writing a report and/or by completing an evaluation sheet on the trainee's progress. This must be documented and discussed in detail with the trainee and signed by both the trainer and the trainee. Importantly this does not necessarily mean that the trainee agrees with the assessment but that he/she has had the opportunity to see and discuss it. Clearly if there is a problem with the assessment then this is an area for discussion with the Programme Director. The trainer will need to ensure that all assessments and reports are documented and signed by both the trainer and trainee.

An area in which most trainers will require support and guidance is in carrying out appraisal and assessment and giving constructive feedback. A Director will need to review regularly these processes to ensure not only that reports are being done but that they are being done appropriately.

Finally trainers will need to inform the Programme Directors of problems with the trainees at an early stage so that a failing trainee can be identified at an early stage.

The responsibility of the neurosurgical trainee

Trainees will need to be aware of an important fact- their training is their responsibility. While a programme may be well designed with trainers who are committed, effective and efficient and a Director committed to training, it is entirely up to the individual trainee to get the best out of their training and, if they do, this will inevitably improve the programme.

Appendix I

Criteria for a neurosurgical training programme director

1. The Director of Training need not be the Head of Department.
2. He/She should be a certified specialist for a minimum of 5 years.
3. He/She should work full-time within the Department(s) central to the Training Programme.
4. The CV of the Director should provide evidence of current and continuing scientific work.
5. An Assistant Director must be appointed and should be a certified specialist for a minimum of 5 years.

6. The Director must have full secretarial and administrative support.
7. Designated time must be allocated to ensure Programme Directors have sufficient protected time to carry out their responsibilities.

Appendix II

Responsibilities of a training programme director

The principal responsibilities include establishing a transparent and fair selection and appointment process for trainees.

After appointment of a trainee a Training Agreement must be completed by the Director and signed by the trainee and the Director. This is an educational contract and should provide the trainee with an overview of his/her training.

The promotion of an ethos of a high level of professional conduct and ethics within the training programme is essential.

To trainees

a. Organise and co-ordinate a fully balanced Training Programme.
b. Monitor, counsel and inform.
c. Ensure trainees attend appropriate and approved courses.
d. Assist and provide leadership for the assessment of trainees on a six monthly basis.
e. Organise trainees appraisal processes.
f. Assess the competence and knowledge of trainees.
g. Ensure Training Portfolios are up to date.
h. Provide valid documentary evidence of the satisfactory completion of training.

To trainers

a. To evaluate the effectiveness of education and academic provision.
b. To ensure that trainers have the appropriate training and support.
c. To ensure that relevant documentation is completed in a timely (contemporaneous) fashion (assessment reports, evaluation sheet, logbooks).
d. To ensure trainers are fulfilling their training obligations.

To the authority responsible for recognition of the training programme

a. To ensure that the Training Programme functions as agreed.
b. Inform the Authority of major changes in facilities, trainers, trainees.
c. Report failing trainees and trainers to the Authority.
d. To organise and prepare their Unit for site inspections.
e. To advise on the facilities needed for training.

Appendix III

Criteria for neurosurgical trainers

1. A Trainer should be a certified specialist.
2. Trainers should be committed to and familiar with the requirements of the Training Programme.
3. Trainers need to recognise their responsibilities and reconcile them with service pressures.
4. Trainers will require secretarial and administrative support.

Responsibilities of neurosurgical trainers

1. Meet at an early stage with the trainee and establish their experience and identify training needs.
2. Set realistic aims and objective for 6 months.
3. Possess the skills to carry out appraisal and assessment and give constructive feedback.
4. Supervise the day to day work of the trainee on the ward, in the clinic and in the operating theatre.
5. Assess trainee's surgical competency on a continual basis.
6. Supervise, check and sign the trainee's log book at regular intervals.
7. At the end of the 6-month-training period assess and report on the trainee's progress(evaluation form).
8. Ensure that all assessments and reports are documented and signed by both the trainer and the trainee.
9. To inform the Programme Director of problems at an early stage.

Correspondence: G. Neil-Dwyer, Wessex Neurological Centre, Southampton University Hospitals, Tremona Road, Southampton SO16 6YD, Hampshire, UK. e-mail: glenn@neil-dwyer.com

Acta Neurochir (2004) [Suppl] 90: 17–19

Printed in Austria

III Teaching staff

J. Lobo Antunes

Serviço de Neurocirurgia, Hospital de Santa Maria, Lisboa, Portugal

Education of a surgeon is a lifelong process where two components can be distinguished: one is what may be called the *formal curriculum* and is analyzed according to the current principles of medical education using a somewhat reductionist and predominantly quantitative approach. It often begins with definition of the educational goals which, in our discipline, are usually aimed at training a "general neurosurgeon". It should be stated, however, that the extent to which it is permissible to demand from those who have just finished their training complete technical autonomy in dealing with the most complex pathologies that constitute general practice in our specialty, is not at all clear. In the United States, residents who have finished a training program usually have to move elsewhere, joining other surgeons in group practices or go to specific areas for additional training. In Europe, in many instances, the "training period" does not end with conclusion of a six-year-program since trainees remain in the same clinical environment for a few additional years. But there is necessarily a fair amount of variation among the different countries in Europe concerning the very definition of the training goals and methodology that is required for its fulfilment.

There is general agreement, however, that there should be a clear definition of a timetable of rotations, of a quota of surgical procedures that may guarantee an acceptable degree of technical competence, a structured learning program which should preferably include a period in a research laboratory, and explicit criteria of evaluation, since any formal curriculum is closely tied to an evaluation process.

When I started to reflect on my own education as a neurosurgeon and searched for the intangible components of this mixture of theoretical knowledge learned from books and from the experiences in my own life, of good and bad examples, courage and cowardice, altruism and egoism, triumph and defeat, I began to appreciate the concept of the "*hidden curriculum*" [1]. This is engraved in the bricks, the mortar, and the memory of a school or a department and is preserved and transmitted from generation to generation. This curriculum is much more difficult to evaluate, as its appraisal slowly emerges within ourselves and gains its voice throughout life. This curriculum takes form in the wards, in the locker room, in the cafeteria, in the operating room, in the emergency room, everywhere we are called to do our job. It has no timetable, gives no credits or diplomas, is often silent or rooted in an oral tradition, and is made up of stories, anecdotes, personal experiences or aphorisms.

The *formal curriculum* is particularly concerned about the training of trainers. The *hidden curriculum* is fed by models [6] which, in their essence, are the purest expression of professional solidarity. Wilder Penfield once wrote that "no man goes alone on his eventful journey through medical school" [3]. Models are defined by qualities that include compassion, sense of humour, integrity, ability to teach, capacity to explain clearly in a non intimidating fashion complex matters, technical competence and tact in our relationship with patients and their families. All this is crucial for a well balanced teaching staff.

I would also like to emphasize that there is much to be learned from non-medical professionals, and during my residency in New York, I learned a lot from the experienced nurses working there. Throughout my life as a neurosurgeon I have learned even more from my patients.

So it is clear to me that the "skeleton" of this hidden curriculum is made up of values that are easy to recognize but hard or even impossible to quantify: sense of duty, curiosity, diligence, integrity and altruism. But it also requires the understanding of ambiguity, uncertainty and error. My point is simply this: education of any physician needs to find a proper balance between two indispensable forms: the *formal* and the *hidden*.

This somewhat long introduction was necessary in my view to put forth what I believe are the crucial issues in the matter I am supposed to discuss – the training staff of a department. I dealt with them already some years ago in the European Lecture of the EANS [2].

The ideal setting for teaching may take different forms. Many of us are convinced that we run nearly perfect services which we strongly dominate by the lustre of our personalities. Alone we can do very little, however, as we need people with various intellectual abilities, technical skills, and scientific interests, and it is the tapestry of interwoven talents and temperaments which constitutes a true *school of surgery*.

A school of surgery needs different actors to play different roles. It requires a *leader* who preferably should be the Chief of Service, who represents the repository of experience, and who should be an acknowledged expert within a specific clinical area. In my view it is important that the "Chief" is someone with an outstanding technical or scientific reputation, a truism which in fact is not always understood.

It is certainly crucial to have among the staff group a "*scientist*", someone who can help to set a research project, to teach the scientific method, to criticize the results, to introduce objectivity and precision into clinical reasoning.

It is equally helpful to have a "*scholar*", and true scholarship is sadly dying out in our profession. He or she will be able to give the correct reference, to teach how to write an article, to make trainees acquainted with the history of our discipline, to develop a sense of healthy scepticism about what they read. This is probably the person who should also be in charge of the "Journal Club" and of the library of the department.

Of course it is also indispensable to have a number of "*teachers of surgery*". Although we all would like to shape artists, the truth is that we have mostly to form artisans. Many of us when working will just move along, not sensing the need to explain, happy to be watched like any great performer. It is true that surgical teaching places emphasis on decision making accounting for about 75% of any operation. This is perhaps one reason why teaching dexterity has been so neglected. Other reasons are that teaching technique is very time consuming and many people don't know how to do it, anyway. So it is absolutely crucial to have people with ability and taste to teach the craft in all its minute details, from the correct position of the patient to the strategic placement of the bone flap. They will show the trainee how to handle the tissues gently and care for the tools with affection. Those, like me, who were fortunate to have had that kind of master will always feel their presence in the operating room, standing behind them observing and guiding.

I believe that it is quite useful to have a "*confessor*", someone the trainees can appeal to to find solace, and upon whose shoulder they can shed their tears. He will absolve the mistakes, confiding that he made them himself, but at the same time assuring that all will end well, even when the situation seems hopeless. They play an irreplaceable stabilizing role, and this is particularly important as it has recently been emphasized by Volpp et al. [5]. It is essential to have a frank discussion of the errors committed, otherwise silence prevails and errors tend to be concealed. In a study by Wu et al. [7] only 54 percent of the house officers told their attending physician about the most serious errors they had committed in the previous year. As noticed, trainees who are willing to accept responsibility for their errors and to discuss them are more likely to report constructive changes in practice than trainees who do not openly acknowledge their errors.

It also helps to have a "*bureaucrat*" in a positive sense of the word, somebody who can help the Chief of the Department often too busy to run the daily teaching affairs. He coordinates the various educational activities, checks the surgical logbook, relates to the hospital officers, organizes and programs the rotations through the various departments, etc. It may be relevant that each trainee has an assigned *tutor*, with whom he may develop a more intimate professional and personal relationship.

I think it is important to emphasize that in a teaching hospital everybody should be involved in the process of teaching and that includes, of course, the trainees themselves. In other words, it is essential that a teaching philosophy permeates the daily activities of a service, and the more advanced resident should assist and help the juniors. In my experience in the United States, this contributed to creating a sense of hierarchy and discipline that was quite useful for the daily running of the service and a growing sense of leadership.

Conclusion

In conclusion, I would like to insist that surgical education should always be a molding process tailored to the needs of each trainee. This requires a teaching staff composed of different personalities and talent. And returning to the concluding remarks from my European Lecture, with all this in mind, we will be prepared to teach and study a profession that still belongs, in the words of Trotter [4], to the "very small class of professions [that] in this tame world can be called jobs for men (...). By it I mean professions in which it is possible for people – men or women – to pursue the dying ideal that an occupation for adults should allow for intellectual freedom, should give character as much chance as cleverness, and should be subject to the tonic of difficulty and the spice of danger."

References

1. Hafferty FW (1998) Beyond curriculum reform: confronting medicine's hidden curriculum. Acad Med 73: 403–407
2. Lobo Antunes J (1987) Teaching and learning neurosurgery. Acta Neurochir (Wien) 86: 69–74
3. Penfield W (1977) No man alone: a neurosurgeon's life. Little Brown, Boston, pp 31–32
4. Trotter W (1946) Art and science in medicine. The collected papers. Oxford University Press, p 85
5. Volpp KGM, Grande D. (2003) Residents' suggestions for reducing errors in teaching Hospitals. N Engl J Med 348: 851–855
6. Wright SM, Kern DE, Kolodener K, Howard DM et al. (1998) Attributes of excellent attending – physician role models. N Engl J Med 339: 1986–1993
7. Wu AW, Folkman S, Mc Phee SI, Lo B. (1991) Do house officers learn from their mistakes? JAMA 265: 2089–2094

Correspondence: J. Lobo Antunes, M.D. Ph.D., Department of Neurosurgery, Hospital Santa Maria, Av. Prof. Egas Moniz, 1649-035 Lisbon, Portugal. e-mail: jlobo.antunes@mail.telepac.pt

Acta Neurochir (2004) [Suppl] 90: 21–31

Printed in Austria

IV The ideal neurosurgical training curriculum

A. General aspects

D. M. Long

Department of Neurosurgery, Johns Hopkins Medicine, Baltimore, USA

Introduction

There are two aspects to the development of an ideal curriculum for neurosurgical training which are fundamental to curriculum structure. Of course, local considerations may change specific sequences so the ideal curriculum is always more theoretical than practical. What is important is not to slavishly follow any guidelines for sequencing material but to understand the concepts of competency-based training as a way to assure the competency of training program graduates and to prepare them for the next phase of postgraduate medical education which leads to mastery of our field [9].

There are some theoretical teaching considerations which underlie the development of any curriculum [7]. Much is known about perceptual learning [1]. The general agreement is that the students learn best through memorization and understanding rules as a first step, followed by externally directed learning, usually in the form of lectures, conferences or core curricula. Then students progress to self-directed learning in which the trainees take primary responsibility for their education with guidance from faculty and mentors. How we learn and how we apply that knowledge are important issues in any educational system. One schema which is particular germane to neurosurgery proposes that we first begin by acquiring necessary skills such as history taking, the neurological examination, interpretation of imaging studies, and how to do procedures. We then learn to apply these skills through following sets of rules first laid down by experts and then developed for ourselves. From rules following the master surgeon should progress to knowledge-based practice in which the product of all knowledge and experience is correctly applied often without a specific sequential thought process [2, 10, 11]. The synthesis of much material has occurred within the brain automatically and is then applied effectively, often without specific steps [4].

There is much information concerning various stages of learning and what it takes to progress from each stage [3]. In surgical training we take beginners with very little previous practical experience in neurosurgery and very little specific neurosurgical information to enter training. From the beginning the goal of neurosurgery training is the progression to competency to practice the field. It is of interest that there is very little information about how long it takes or what kind of application is required in terms of hours of training and practice to move from the beginning stage to competency [5]. Much more is known about the next phase in which the competent practitioner progresses to mastery of the field. Comparison of a number of diverse occupations indicates that it takes about ten thousand hours of practice and approximately ten years to move to clear mastery of a field. Therefore we have to always remember that the training program has a twin goal of producing a competent practitioner and preparing that practitioner for self-directed education which leads to the desired goal of master surgeon. Core curricula are fundamental to a competency-based training program, but in themselves do not represent competency. In order to become competent it is necessary to know the body of skills and knowledge which define competency. The American College of Surgeons, The American Association of Neurological Surgeons/Congress of Neurological Surgeons, and the Society of Neurological Surgeons have all developed core curricula for different phases of training. Whenever a curriculum is developed there is then a great tendency to treat that information as the maximum which is to be learned. In fact, core curricula always should represent the minimum and only lead the perceptual learner through externally directed learning. The next phase of self-directed learning is key to development of competency and for progressing to mastery after competency [10].

There is one other concept which is important to think about. How material to be learned is presented is very important. In the first phases of perceptual learning when memorization and rules following are important, it is essential to have didactic presentations which present both the minimum material to be learned and the rules to be followed. This can be achieved for example by rules presenting how the information should be applied to obtain a desirable outcome most of the time. However, these formal presentations have little value once learning becomes self-directed. There is good information that they do not impart new information effectively. The traditional lectures, grand rounds presentations, teaching conferences conducted only by senior neurosurgeons, and all other non-participatory conferences have limited impact on education, and cannot prepare the trainee for lifelong learning [10].

The ideal training program year by year

Ideally I believe that the concept of numbered post-graduate years should be eliminated and all students should progress within the neurosurgery training program as rapidly as their individual skills and acquisition of knowledge allow. However, we have to start somewhere in making a transition so it is reasonable to use the current post graduate year (PGY) concept as a format (Table 1). We should realize that in an ideal training program these designations should have no meaning. Rather we should think about what needs to be learned, what applications are required, and what independent judgements the trainee should be able to exercise. These are likely to be sequenced according to local needs and patterns of practice rather than conform to any idealized program. What is important is that the core curricula be mastered at a minimum and that residents proceed in training with escalating responsibilities as rapidly as their individual skills allow.

Table 1. *The current Johns Hopkins residency program*

PGY 1	12 months	General Surgery, Neurology (3 mos), Surgical Specialties
PGY 2	12 months	General, Tumor, Vascular, Spine Neurosurgery
PGY 3	12 months	Pediatrics, Functional, General Neurosurgery
PGY 4	12 months	Chief Residency, 4 months of each- Tumor, Vascular, Spine
PGY 5, 6	24 months	Required Research Training
PGY 7	12 months	Supervised Practice- 4 months each of Tumor, Vascular, Spine, Subspecialization

The current training program

PGY 1-the internship

What do trainees need to learn in the internship as it currently is structured in the United States? Trainees need to learn conduct in the operating room and fundamental operative skills. They need to understand fluid and electrolyte balance and nutrition. They should become familiar with the management of patients suffering trauma. They should learn to recognize and treat surgical complications and they should have experience in those surgical specialities which are most inter-related with neurosurgical practice later. In the United States it has been decided that the neurology experience should also occur in the first year. I personally do not believe that three months of neurology in the first year of training is sufficient to provide the ideal of the surgical neurologist which was a part of the founding concept of neurosurgery. However, it is quite reasonable that the management of stroke, central nervous system infections, and neurological intensive care all be learned in the first year. Extensive experience in general surgery beyond what is needed to master fundamental surgical skills is not required and there is little educational purpose to extended periods of patient care dealing with diseases which are not pertinent to neurosurgery. PGY 1 has been modified to provide six months of general surgery and 6 months of neurology/surgical specialties.

PGY 2, 3, 4

Current requirements in the United States are for 36 additional months of clinical training in neurosurgery.[1] These 36 months must culminate in a chief residency in which quasi-independent practice is possible. Of course, legal requirements mean that this experience can never truly be independent. In our training program we have broken down the 36 months into junior residency (12months), senior residency (12months), and chief residency (12months). In most training programs of the past there was very little sub-specialization and assignments were generally made on the basis of assisting individual surgeons or general experience in a specific hospital. Sub-specialty practice is now common in academic centers and in larger group practices throughout the world. Training programs should reflect this trend to sub-specialization. Since the concept of junior and senior resident disappears in a competency-based program it is not necessary to stratify training. Thus for the 24 months required before chief residency we now assign residents according to broad sub-specialty categories. These include: 1. Tumor neurosurgery 2. Vascular neurosurgery 3. Surgery of the spine 4. Pediatric neurosurgery (including pediatric trauma) 5. Peripheral nerve surgery 6. Pain 7. Functional neurosurgery including stereotaxis for all purposes 8. Epilepsy surgery. At Johns Hopkins trauma is not a separate service and trauma experience is primarily in pediatrics and spread throughout the residency.

In addition we have one affiliated hospital which is a general hospital. A general practice of neurosurgery which is not specialized is the core of the experience in this affiliate.

In addition residents return for at least one month of neurological intensive care to supplement the two-three month experience of the first year.

Tumor, vascular, and spinal neurosurgery are experienced twice during the 24 month period. All of the other rotations are a single experience. All these rotations are currently of a specific length and content.

It is the responsibility of the director of each service to define for the trainees what should be learned in terms of knowledge and skills. Knowledge is assessed by an examination at the end of each rotation. At present the assessment of skills and the application of both skills and knowledge is left to the judgement of the faculty. We currently have no better way and there is good evidence that the judgement of experts is reliable [12]. In the ideal program no resident should complete one of these rotations without having satisfactorily demonstrated competence in all of the minimum skills defined by the faculty. Furthermore they should progress beyond these minimums as rapidly and as far as their personal abilities allow. By defining the sequence of skills acquisition in the operating room and allowing the residents to move ahead independently in applying these skills we demonstrated acceleration of competency to do specific neurosurgical operations by 6 to 18 months. This strongly suggests that our current training programs retard the speed with which many residents can progress in training. In competency-based training residents should move ahead as rapidly as they demonstrate competency and this simply means moving from one set of skills to another so that much more is learned for any given period of assignment. No resident should complete one of these rotations until all the faculty involved agree that competency has been gained in at least the minimum skills defined as the requirement of the rotation [8, 9, 10].

The core curricula which underlie these rotations are being developed from a variety of sources. The specific sequence in which material is learned is going to vary from institution to institution. What is important is that the minimums should be uniform throughout the world and that residents should have the opportunity to pass beyond the minimums as rapidly as their individual talents allow.

There is another fundamental premise in the idea of competency-based training. Residents should be able to make independent patient management judgements when they are deemed competent to do so and the independence of these judgements should escalate according to experience and demonstrated competence. In today's legal environment in the United States it is not possible for residents to truly function independently but they should be given the ability to demonstrate that they could be independent at each level before competency is verified [10].

PGY 4 – the chief residency

Chief residency experience is now 12 months. During that time residents are expected to take on major responsibilities for evaluation of patients, implementation of treatment plans, and the surgical experience. This traditional training concept of quasi-indepen-

[1] According to the European Training Charter a minimum of 4 years must be spent in clinical neurosurgery. The curriculum can be organized appropriately. (H.J.R.)

dence which has been fundamental in the United States for the past hundred years is under attack from the legal profession, but persists as a requirement for certification. Independent practice is not possible so supervision must occur in ways that assure patient safety without compromising the educational experience for chief residents. During the chief residency trainees should have the opportunity to examine patients independently without being influenced by the prior information from senior neurosurgeons. The training program should require that they develop treatment plans including prognosis and treatment alternatives, interact with patients, participate in surgical procedures to the extent of their abilities, and do all of this in a progressively escalating fashion in which they achieve greater and greater independence throughout the year. This should culminate in complete independence. Specific numbers of operative procedures are not required in American training programs. There are minimums for number of craniotomies, and examining board members and residency reviews make arbitrary judgements about the adequacy of numbers of procedures done, but there are no specified numbers required, and therefore the experience of chief residents may vary enormously from one training program to another. Our trainees at Johns Hopkins typically have 350–500 operations in the chief year. Training to competency is the goal of the chief year. Now we clearly define the end of training as that degree of competency which will allow independent practice the following year without endangering patients. This means that every chief resident must be competent to do most procedures of neurosurgery. Remember competency does not imply mastery [10]. Competency means that the individual will carry out all aspects of patient care at the level of his or her peers and in a fashion that does not endanger patients. It does not imply that every trainee will be a master of every field or that every trainee can do everything in neurosurgery irrespective of how difficult it may be. Competency means that individuals can practice independently while knowing their own limitations, and that they are prepared for the ongoing education which will lead to mastery of those parts of neurosurgery he/she chooses to emphasize. I do not believe that competency can be assured by exposure to specific numbers of patients, by independent practice without supervision, by observation without experience, or through acquisition of a knowledge base alone.

A year of supervised practice

For many years at Johns Hopkins we have supplemented traditional residency training with a year of supervised, though independent, practice as originally envisioned by Halstead [7]. After completion of training for the required 48 months of neurosurgery all Johns Hopkins trainees stay one additional year serving as *instructors* in the medical school and independent members of the faculty. This year supplements the traditional chief residency with a year of busy practice in which trainees maintain independent clinics, evaluate patients, plan treatment, provide prognosis, carry out surgery, and administer all peri-operative care. They are required to verify all of this information with senior faculty in the pertinent sub-specialties and senior faculty members serve as assistants during virtually all surgical procedures. A typical year of independent practice sees the trainee adding about 350–400 major neurosurgical operations to their experience. Sub-specialization is possible, if desired, and may substitute for a fellowship year.

Fellowship years

It is now a common practice for trainees to progress from residency to fellowships in specialized areas of neurosurgery. I personally believe that the introduction of true competency-based training concepts will allow the enfolding of much specialty training into our current programs. As residents accelerate learning and skills application, they will progress to areas of sub-specialization more rapidly. I think this will reduce the amount of time required for post-graduate subspecialty training. It is my view that competency to practice a sub-specialty should be demonstrated in the same way that competencies are assessed throughout residency program and should not be dependent upon time spent in fellowship training. Rather it is the acquisition and application of knowledge and skills which should define sub-specialty competency [12].

Laboratory training

Board requirements in the United States now include one year of research experience. There is very strong evidence that very few neurosurgeons continue research, and it is my view that research training should become an elective as any other sub-specialty. At Johns Hopkins we have had a 2 year requirement for research for many years. I believe that all neurosurgeons would benefit from an experience in clinical research which could be possibly as short as one year. It is unlikely that even 2 years of laboratory research are enough to prepare the trainee for competitive research, and those who wish to do bench research as a part of their career should have the opportunity to be adequately prepared. Such preparation might involve 3 or more years of training. The possibility of a Ph.D. experience should be a part of neurosurgery training. However, these options should be available only for those who wish to take advantage of them and there is little value in all trainees continuing to receive basic research training.

Close reading, statistical methods, study design, and the related issues can be taught to competency by specific programs rather than learned haphazardly in the course of less structured research training. Clinical research training would be of value for all neurosurgeons. I believe basic research training should be limited to those with a serious interest in pursuing research as a part of an academic career and that training should be expanded beyond what is currently available. An obligatory year of basic research serves little educational purpose [6].

Professionalism

The competent practice of medicine requires certain behavioral patterns which are loosely termed professionalism. These include relations with and dedication to patients, relations with peers, meeting documentation standards, personal behavior that never compromises patient care, and a dedication to life-long learning as examples. There is excellent evidence that students and residents who deviate from standards of professional behavior often have difficulty in practice and are disciplined frequently. No one knows how to impart these ideals of professional behavior but excellent mentors are thought to be extremely important. In today's complex medical practice it is also important that didactic educational programs which detail the many administrative responsibilities of physicians are presented to trainees.

Case management as an educational technique

The traditional didactic forums in residency training are Grand Rounds which usually are in lecture form, patient conferences in which ad hoc presentations are the rule, pathology and radiology conferences where ad hoc review of recent cases is carried out, walking rounds which depend upon the nature of hospitalized patients, and journal clubs which review important current papers. All of these forms have significant short-comings though all are valuable for different reasons.

The *formal lecture* is most valuable to the person giving it for all need to learn how to synthesize material, to present it effectively, and to incorporate visual aides for teaching purposes. A summary lecture given by an expert can present material not easily available in any other way. However, when conferences are not participatory they are unlikely to be remembered, and an emphasis upon lectures as an educational form probably retards the acquisition of knowledge. *Patient conferences* and *rounds* which are ad hoc suffer from the fact they are not comprehensive or rank ordered by importance, and typically do not expose the trainee to the spectrum of diseases. *Didactic conferences* in neuro-pathology and neuro-radiology have the same problems if they depend upon current patients for material and can be better organized if they are comprehensive and sequential. *Journal clubs* are of value if they teach close reading, study design, assessment of statistical treatments, and look seriously at the value of the reports being reviewed. If they simply substitute for reading current literature they have little merit.

Case management conferences offer a significant improvement over the conventional forms and are particularly amenable to computerization and standardization. In an appropriately designed case management format patients are sequentially presented beginning with the most typical and progressing to the most unusual presentations of any specific disease. Diagnostic possibilities are outlined; prognosis is determined; alternative therapies described and the outcomes of these therapies presented; moral, ethical and research issues where pertinent can be included. I believe that development of fundamental case management system covering all of neurosurgical disease will be an extremely important next step in educational evolution. The organization of these conferences is also important. They should be participatory and symposium in style. The patient should be presented and the trainees challenged to make the appropriate diagnosis based upon history and physical examination, to interpret the imaging and other diagnostic studies, and to discuss therapeutic options and their outcomes. (See also chapter P. Winkler/J. C. Tonn)

There is also excellent evidence that individuals remember and synthesize material best if it is repeated multiple times and if it is encountered in multiple venues. Neurosurgical trainees should encounter a broad spectrum of diseases in the clinic. A lack of clinic experience is a major deficit in neurosurgical training throughout the world currently. Trainees will then encounter the same problems in the hospital, in the intensive care unit, and in the operating rooms, as well as through related case management conferences. This combination of approaches improves retention and recall [10].

Clinic experience

The issue of clinic experience is an extremely important one. Increasingly in the United States, all surgical specialties find their training focused upon inpatients who come to surgery or suffer significant complications. In most diseases there will be large numbers of patients who do not come to surgery. Some patients will not even have the disease as suspected. The outcome of procedures can only be known with long-term follow-up and trainees are usually excluded from this follow-up. It is extremely important that trainees have a defined outpatient experience which parallels their operative experience and escalates in responsibility in the same way that procedural skills do. This outpatient experience can be correlated with formal case management training to provide a much broader analysis of disease than is possible when one focuses only upon inpatients who are having procedures.

Summary

The current training program at Johns Hopkins is 7 years in length. The first year is equally divided by general surgery and neurology/neurosurgery-related sub-specialties. This year needs to be restructured so that it meets all the specific education required by the beginning neurosurgeon.

In our program the next three years are spent in residency escalating from junior to senior to chief resident to complete the additional required 36 months of training for board eligibility. It is this phase of training that is most amenable to change through competency-based teaching. No one knows how long this residency training should be, and there is very little information about how rapidly neurosurgeons can acquire the requisite knowledge and skills to practice independently. It is important that these years escalate in responsibility and culminate in supervised quasi-independent practice. It is my belief that with escalation based upon demonstrated competencies most residents will progress through training much faster then they do currently. This will allow enfolding of much sub-speciality training into existing programs, especially in the chief year [10].

Years 5 and 6 at Johns Hopkins are spent in a required laboratory rotation though clinical research and sub-specialization which leads to a certification have been reasonable alternatives. It is my belief that obligatory laboratory time serves little useful purpose for most residents. I think basic laboratory research should be reserved for the small number of neurosurgeons who are actually committed to a research career. Most neurosurgeons would benefit from participation in structured clinical research. Research should be treated like any other sub-specialty rather than viewed as a requirement in my opinion.

The final required year at Johns Hopkins has been spent as a faculty member with an independent but supervised practice. This is the key year for competency training in my opinion. Trainees should be allowed to sub-specialize as they continue to expand experience in all fields. This year may be enough to meet any sub-specialty requirements if those are defined by competencies rather than by time. Our residents consider this final year the most important to their successful training and I believe the concept of a final year of supervised practice should be expanded to become a requirement in all training programs. It is in this final year that the acquisition of all competencies should be proven for certification.

An ideal training program utilizes competency as the measure of progression through the program and ignores years in training. The acquisition of knowledge is emphasized progressively to self-directed learning. The application of skills should be carefully monitored from rules following to knowledge-based practice and educational techniques should reflect individual learning styles and the new information available to direct perceptual learning. In the ideal training program the core of knowledge and skills required for each aspect of neurosurgery is defined in advance. Beginners are guided by external directed learning techniques through the minimums to self-directed learning which should occur at whatever rate each trainee can accomplish. Skills are acquired in the same way and no trainee should advance through the training program without demonstrated mastery of the minimums of both knowledge and skills at each level. These concepts mean major changes in our training programs. Education becomes the focus of training and service is relegated to those issues which support the educational mission. That does not mean that service ceases to exist. A part of the educational mission is giving senior faculty members time to teach. However, it does mean that service alone is not a justification for any trainee activity. Trainees will have to demonstrate that acquired skills can be applied effectively at levels deemed acceptable by expert practitioners of neurosurgery. No one will complete any part of a training program without having demonstrated both the knowledge and the skills sufficient to assure competency required for that level [10].

National and international verification of competency is important. Knowledge can be assessed by written examination and is done so quite well now in the United States. Skills are probably best judged by other expert practitioners in the field. The application of knowledge can be assessed by case management techniques. If we are really going to be serious about examining the application of knowledge we need to develop much better methods than the current brief oral ad hoc assessment by our board examinations. This is a field where computerized standard examinations have enormous promise for assessment and educational purposes. Still careful evaluation of application of knowledge and skills by personal contact with master neurosurgeons must remain a part of the assessment process.

Competency-based training offers an enormous opportunity for research in neurosurgical education and in how to assess competency. Self-assessment should be a part of the requirements for every training program, and for every neurosurgeon. Outcomes will eventually be used to define training programs and the practice of their trainees. Competency-based training focuses upon product, not process, so competency, not years of training, becomes the goal.

The original goal of the liberal education was to prepare students to be responsible citizens. Our own training programs are in danger of becoming purely technical. As we change to competency as the primary goal of residency training, we must assure that the liberal aspects of that training are also improved. Deviation to patient welfare, lifelong learning, and effective neurosurgery citizenship all characterize the competent neurosurgeon who will proceed to mastery of the field. Assuring all those desirable characteristics of professionalism is another challenge of competency-based training.

B. Curriculum development in neurosurgery

Introduction

The goal of neurosurgery training is the assurance of competency. Therefore, the first step has to be to understand what is meant by competency in order to define what it will take to make the aspiring neurosurgeon competent. Competency has a specific definition within a theoretical framework. The categories generally accepted are Novice, Beginner, Advanced Beginner, and Competent, beyond competency stand Expert and Master. In general terms we can think of these categories as they relate to the current concept of post-graduate years in training (PGY). Year 1, or the internship, is the Novice year, year 2 is the Beginner year, years 3 and 4 are the Advanced Beginner years and the progression of understanding responsibility and skills should bring the trainee from Advanced Beginner in year 2 to Competent by the end of year 4. These goals are summarized in Table A. A competent physician should have the knowledge, surgical techniques, and patient management skills adequate to practice independent neurosurgery, be prepared for lifetime learning, and be prepared to mature to Expert and Master of the field over the next 10 to 20 years. The program must define the knowledge required, examine the application of that knowledge, define the surgical skills required and assess proficiency, and

Table A.

What must be done to assure Competency

1. Define competency?
   A. Knowledge
   B. Application of knowledge
   C. Skills (Surgical Proficiency)
   D. Application of Skills

The competent physician should manage patients and their problems at a level expected of others of equivalent experience.

2. Define the knowledge and skills required and the sequence of learning
3. Define measurement of competency
4. Develop the curriculum
5. Define outcome measures

Table B.

1. Medical Knowledge
2. Patient Care- Application of Knowledge
3. Medical Skills
4. Procedural Skills
5. Application of Skills to Patient Care
6. Practice Improvement- Use of Texts and Literature- Self-Directed Learning
7. Interpersonal and Communication Skills
8. Professionalism

determine the application of those skills to patient care. In addition, this sequence of acquisition must be determined independently for each training program. Organized neurosurgery should define measures of competence, devise a minimum core curriculum, and examine outcome measures for the educational process.

General competencies

There are a group of general competencies that every physician must have and every neurosurgical trainee certainly must acquire these skills. These are listed in Table B. The training program has to assess technical competency to perform procedures and the application of knowledge and surgical skills to patient care on a continuous basis. Progress and acquisition of knowledge can be assessed by written or oral examination such as those used by the American Board of Neurological Surgery. It is important to assess professional behavior and require moral, ethical, and personal competence in all aspects of professionalism throughout training.

Surgical skills curriculum

Acquisition of surgical skills should be sequenced from least complex to most complex and sequenced throughout the training program. Table C demonstrates the general progression. The sequence actual procedures can be determined independently in each program in accordance with the overall goals of the curriculum.

Table C.

1. Assisting a qualified surgeon until knowledge of anatomy and instrument use is verified.
2. Positioning and Preparing
3. Closure
4. Opening and Exposure
5. Progressively performing the procedure with supervision
6. Independent Surgery

Table D.

1. The Doctor- Patient Relationship
2. Conduct of Medical Research
3. Valid Study Design and Research
4. Responsible Medical Writing/Speaking
5. Communicating with Patients
6. Close Reading, Critical Thinking
7. Conflict of Interest
8. Relations with Peers
9. Quality Assurance and Outcomes Assessment
10. Physician Impairment and Discipline

Professionalism in the ideal curriculum

Teaching neurosurgery trainees to be good doctors, good colleagues, and exemplary human beings is important. This is probably best done by example and mentors who behave correctly are the most important influences for young physicians. Some aspects of professionalism can be taught and discussed in a formal way. Table D lists some of these more important aspects of professional behavior.

The ideal curriculum

Specific curriculum development is being addressed by a number of professional organizations in the United States. The American College of Surgeons and the Society of Neurological Surgeons both have major efforts and core curricula are available or soon will be to supplement those already proposed by our national neurosurgery organizations.

The educational requirements of the Novice (PGY-1) year are found in Table E. During this year the neurosurgical trainees should learn the fundamentals of operative and peri-operative care. They should learn how to deal with the major complications which beset neurosurgery and they should be able to deal with serious multi-system trauma. This is a good time to learn the fundamentals of neurology, particularly acute care neurology. The goal of the year is to prepare the young neurosurgeon with all of the fundamentals which will be needed as the trainee becomes involved exclusively with neurosurgical patients.

Table E. *The ideal curriculum – year one**

1. Peri-operative Evaluation and Management
2. Management of Pain
3. Management of Cardiac Disease
4. Management of Pulmonary Disease
5. Principles of Fluid Balance and Nutrition
6. Cardiopulmonary Resuscitation
7. Fundamental Surgical Skills
8. Fundamentals of Neurology
9. Principles of Acute Care Management
   - Acute Neurological Deterioration
   - Pulmonary Distress
   - Anesthetic Emergencies
   - Multi-system Trauma
   - Coma and Stroke

(See the core curriculum details available from the American College of Surgeons for all recommendations).

Table F. *The ideal curriculum – years two and three general beginning competencies*

1. Fundamentals of Neuro Imaging
2. The Neurological Examination
3. Acute Neurological Deterioration
4. Spinal Emergencies
5. Peripheral Nerve Injury and Repair
6. Principles of Neuroanesthesia

During the Beginner and Advanced Beginner phases of training (PGY-2,3) the trainee becomes exclusively involved in neurological issues. The fundamentals which should be mastered early in the beginning phase are found in Table F. Obviously all of these will be expanded during the entire neurosurgery training. But these topics should all be covered in the first few months of the first year of specific neurosurgery training.

Core curriculum

A draft core curriculum has been presented to the Society of Neurological Surgeons. I present one of these proposals as an example of how a core curriculum should be structured initially. There are two important issues to remember. The first is that the core curriculum is the minimum not the maximum required and the second is that the core curriculum is simply for the introduction of these topics. It is expected that each topic will be developed as a continuum of learning throughout the next three years of training.

There is another important point for all core curricula. They can be as specific or as broad as thought appropriate by each individual program director. The sequence in which these topics are introduced will also be program specific and will vary from program to core program according to the types of patients seen. The topics can be equally broad or specifically defined. The program director may choose to list everything an individual is supposed to know while another may define only broad categories and let the trainees develop the specifics themselves. The importance of the core curriculum lies in the fact that every general topic to be mastered is listed. The general sequence in which these topics should be studied and mastered is defined. The core curriculum should have some relationship to the patient management and surgical experience of the trainee. However, individual programs should take much responsibility for developing their own curricula and integrating the curricula available from organized sources into a curriculum specifically developed for their own purposes. General examples of core curricula are found in Table G sub-topics I–VIII.

General principles of education in patient care

Education in patient care is extremely important. The general principles to be followed are found in Table H. The most important issue is that large numbers of patients must be seen in multiple venues and that trainees must be given the responsibility of formulating independent patient management schema.

Education to competency

The principle of education to competency will eventually eliminate the concept of specific years of postgraduate training. However, in order to make the transition it is necessary to use the PGY concept to have some structure in which the acquisition and application of knowledge can be judged. It is to be expected that with time training programs will gradually change to allow trainees to proceed at their individual rate in both acquisition of knowledge, mastery of surgerical skills, and the application of both to the management of patients with neurosurgical diseases.

Table G. *Curriculum topics-years two and three**

Trauma

1. Head trauma
   - Diagnostic and surgical management of depressed skull fractures
   - Diagnostic and surgical management of acute and chronic subdural hematomas
   - Diagnostic and surgical management of epidural hematomas
   - Diagnostic and surgical management of intracerebral hematomas
   - Management of increased intracranial pressure including ICP measurement
   - Management of DAI and cerebral contusion
   - General trauma management
   - Management of CSF otorrhea and rhinorrhea
   - Recognition of brain death including legal implications
   - Familiarity with AANS/CNS guidelines for management of severe head injury
2. Spine trauma
   - Diagnostic and surgical management of cervical spine injuries
   - Diagnostic and surgical management of thoracic spine injuries
   - Diagnostic and surgical management of lumbar and sacral injuries
   - Fundamental instrumentation techniques
3. Peripheral nerve trauma
   - Recognition and initial management of peripheral nerve trauma
   - Major nerve exploration and repair

Vascular disease

1. Extracranial vascular disease
   - Extra and intracranial occlusive disease
   - Carotid endarterectomy
   - Management of acute infarction and TIA
2. Intracranial vascular disease
   - Intracerebral hematomas
   - Anterior circulation aneurysms
   - Straight forward AVMs
   - Dissections
   - Cavernous malformations
   - Vasospasm management

Tumors

- All glial tumors
- Convexity meningiomas
- Parasellar Tumors
- Neuronavigation
- Cortical localization
- All metastatic tumors
- Pituitary Tumors – functional and nonfunctional

Spine

- Diagnosis and management of degenerative disease
- Management of epidural tumors and infection
- Management of bone infection
- Management of intradural extra axial tumors
- Management of intra axial tumors
- Management of dural AVM
- Basic stabilizing instrumentation

Table G (continued)

Peripheral nerve and functional

- Diagnosis and surgical management of upper and lower extremity compression syndromes
- Diagnosis and management of peripheral nerve tumors
- Diagnosis of Brachial plexus tumors, compressive syndromes and inflammatory disease
- Balloon compression or radiofrequency Rx of trigeminal neuralgia
- Dorsal column stimulator
- MVD for trigeminal neuralgia or other cranial neuralgias
- Cordotomy
- Drug delivery pump (intrathecal)
- Vagal nerve stimulator for seizures
- Temporal lobectomy for seizures
- Sterotactics
- Epilepsy Surgery

Pediatrics and shunting

- Medical and surgical management of common congenital abnormalities
- Medical and surgical management of common brain tumors
- All cranial trauma
- All shunts

Other skills

- Ventriculostomy
- Tongs application
- Halo application
- Muscle and nerve biopsy
- Lumbar CSF drainage and LP
- Peripheral nerve blocks

Skull base surgery

- Acoustic tumors
- Basal meningiomas
- Other skull base training
- Complex approaches to the skull base

*Tables G-I–VIII are a synopsis of draft recommendations presented to the Society of Neurological Surgeons, 2003.

Table H.

1. Large numbers of diverse patients
2. Multiple venues: clinic, ward, emergency, operating room
3. Independent assessment and formulation of management plan
4. Interaction with senior faculty to critique management
5. Large diverse surgical volume
6. Repetition

References

1. Anderson JR (ed) (1981) Cognitive skills and their acquisition. Lawrence Erlbaum, Hillsdale NJ
2. Blum BI, Sigilliot VG (1986) An expert system for designating information systems. Johns Hopkins APL Tech Dig; 7: 23–31
3. Edelman S, Intratar N (2002) Models of perceptual learning. chap. 18 n Perceptual Learning (eds) Poggio and Fahle MIT Press, Campbridge, London
4. Hamill BW, Stewart RI (1986) Modeling the acquisition and representation of knowledge for distributing tactical decision making. Johns Hopkins APL Tech Dig 17:31–38

5. Harden RM, Hart IR, Mulholland H (eds) (1992) Current developments in assessing clinical competence. Page Brothers, Norwich, England
6. Herbert RS, Levine RB, Smith CG, Wright SM (2003) A systematic review of resident research curricula. Acad Med 78 (1): 61–67
7. Long DM (1996) Educating neurosurgeons for the 21st century. Neurosurg Quart 62 (2): 78–88
8. Long DM (1998) Assurance of competency in residency training: neurosurgical education in the 21st Century. Neurosurgery in transition. The socioeconomic transformation of neurological surgery, concepts in neurosurgery, vol 9. In: Bean JR (ed) Williams & Wilkins, Chap 10, 99: 147–156
9. Long DM (2001) Competency based residency training: the next advance in graduate medical education. Risk control and quality management in neurosurgery. In: Steiger HJ, Uhl E (eds) Acta Neurochir (Wien) [Suppl] 78: 153–158
10. Long DM (2004) Competency based training in neurosurgery: the next revolution in medical education. Surg Neurol 61 (1): 5–15
11. Rasmussen J, Lind M (1982) A model of human decision making in complex systems and its use for design of system control strategies. Riso National Laboratory Report. Riso-M-2349. Roskilde, Denmark
12. Williams RG et al (1987) Direct, standardized assessment of clinical competence. Med Educ 21: 482–489

Correspondence: Donlin M. Long, Department of Neurosurgery, Johns Hopkins Medicine, 600 North Wolfe Str./Carnegie 466, Baltimore, MD 21287-7709, USA. e-mail: dmlong@jhmi.edu

Acta Neurochir (2004) [Suppl] 90: 33–38

Printed in Austria

V Internal regulations and general guidelines of a neurosurgical department and training programme

H.-J. Reulen[1] and **H.-J. Steiger**[2]

[1] Department of Neurosurgery, Ludwig-Maximilians-University, Munich, Germany
[2] Department of Neurosurgery, Heinrich-Heine University, Düsseldorf, Germany

Summary

It is strongly recommended that general guidelines and internal regulations be laid down in written form by the department. The guidelines regulate the general workflow and related trainee duties and responsibilities, education and research, special procedures for particular diseases and conditions (standards of care). Regarding general workflow of the department, the following items should be laid down once in written form: time table of department, working hours, admission procedures, medical records directives, responsibilities on wards and in the emergency unit, patient information, discharge procedures, outpatient consultations, call schedule and on-call duty plan, as well as week-end and holiday regulations for rounds on wards and ICU. Regarding education and research, the following items should be written down: conferences and teaching rounds, policies on presentations and publications, policies regarding meetings and courses, research leave and vacation plan. The written definition of standards of care is still considered optional in neurosurgery at the present time.

Keywords: Neurosurgical training programme; regulations and procedures; residency training; standards of care; quality management.

Introduction

It is strongly recommended that internal regulations and general guidelines of a department be laid down in written form. Defined procedures and punctuality are necessary for an efficient workflow and to ensure principal standards in patient care, last but not least also from a medico-legal point of view. Written procedures are the heart of any quality management system. Such "internal regulations" also facilitate daily life and collaboration among doctors, nurses, and other personnel. It is important that a new trainee receives a written hand-out when entering the programme.

This chapter has been designed as a possible guide for all those departments that have not yet developed such internal regulations. It is based on experiences of many years and simultaneously is a collection of good examples seen over the years in different departments. The model presented here in the following sections can either be used as they are or be modified and adjusted to the local situation. Some references are given for further reading.

Internal regulations and guidelines of the department objectives of the training programme

The goal of a training programme is to bring the rising generation efficiently to the necessary level of competent patient care and conduction of scientific research to produce a small group of fine clinicians and scientists. The programme needs trainees who are interested in becoming outstanding clinicians and surgeons devoted to patient care, who are also interested in acquiring basic laboratory and/or clinical research skills that will allow them to contribute to new knowledge and future developments. The training programme emphasises a team approach in the major areas of our specialty. The programme expects outstanding performance from every trainee and in return we are committed to provide an outstanding educational environment for our trainees. The training programme constitutes essentially a contract between two generations of neurosurgeons. The younger generation helps to run the service and receives in exchange devoted formation by the older generation.

List of guidelines

The following items should be laid down once in written form and be revised from time to time. They should be handed to the resident when entering the programme.

A) Workflow and related trainee duties and responsibilities
   1) time table of department
   2) working hours
   3) admission procedures
   4) medical records directives
   5) responsibilities on wards and in the emergency unit
   6) patient information
   7) discharge procedures
   8) outpatient consultations
   9) call schedule and on-call duty plan
   10) weekend and holiday regulation for rounds on wards and ICU

B) Education and research
   1) conferences, teaching rounds and education
   2) presentations and publications
   3) policies regarding meetings and courses
   4) research leave
   5) vacation policies and plan

C) Special management guidelines (standards of care, optional)

In the following examples are given for some of the items from the given table of contents. They can be modified and adjusted to the local situation. Local circumstances determine whether certain concepts can be implemented or not. For example, in our opinion the teaching effect of the educational conferences is optimal if an entire morning of the week is devoted completely to teaching, possibly in combination with ward rounds with the chairman. No elective procedures are planned for this weekday. Implementation of this concept is only possible if the operating theatres are shared with other disciplines to allow for an even utilisation of these resources. Not all items mentioned in the survey are covered.

Workflow and related trainee duties and responsibilities

1. Time Table of Department
Punctuality is critical for efficient functioning of the service

a) *Morning rounds [7, 9]*: Monday to Friday, beginning at (07^{00}) hrs with the respective staff members/consultants.
b) *Morning conference [4]*: Monday to Friday, beginning at (07^{45}) hrs in the conference room.[a] A short report of emergencies and admissions during the night is presented by the trainee on call, a status report on patients of the ICU and intermediate ward by the respective residents, particular occurrences and problems on the wards are reported by the ward residents.
c) *Operating theatres*: OR begin at (08^{15}) hrs according to the OP programme of the day. The surgeon or the assigned trainee must be present in the OR for positioning. Any changes in the OP programme must be made known to the anaesthesiologist and the responsible scrub nurse in due time.
d) *Neuroradiological conference and/or OP conference* Monday to Friday at (14^{00}) hrs in conference room. All newly admitted patients are presented with previous radiological examinations etc., so that the patient management can be planned conclusively, if possible. All patients to be operated the following day are discussed regarding the surgical approach and details of the procedure.
e) *Afternoon ward rounds* (if any)
f) *Intensive care round*: Surgeons must see their patients on the ICU at least once per day and discuss the treatment protocol with the responsible colleagues.[b] Notes are to be written on all neurosurgical ICU patients either by the surgeon or by the trainee.
g) *Briefing of trainee on call*: Important information shall be transmitted to the trainee on call within the frame of a formal transfer. A list of all patients has to be generated to update the trainee on call on the status of all patient problems on the service.

Working hours[c]

Admission procedures

a) Patients are admitted either to the department in general or to one of the consultants/staff specifi-

[a] Most European departments have morning conferences where all staff members and trainees participate.

[b] The personal care by the designated attending surgeon is a traditional concept in the USA. In Europe the personal care by the responsible surgeon is also the concept which meets best the expectations of the patients and relatives. Furthermore, specific knowledge of the details of the pathology and the surgical procedure is necessary for an appropriate assessment and management of surgical ICU patients.

[c] There is no general standard for the working hours and changes are to be expected in the light of new European and national regulations. Still, it is advisable to define the working hours and also the dependence of working hours on specific needs of the patients and the department [5].

cally. Patients in the outpatient clinic are seen by the assigned trainee together with the respective consultant/staff.

b) Patients arriving directly on the ward are seen by the assigned trainee as soon as possible. History taking, physical examination, and the organisation of further laboratory, radiological or – if necessary – additional examinations are indispensably required on day of admission. All patients should have a full physical and neurological examination and a documented plan for necessary lab and x-ray work-up. New admissions are to be discussed with the respective consultant/staff and the further procedure is determined.

c) Emergencies admitted through the emergency unit are seen by the trainee on call, who discusses the case and further procedures after primary assessment with the consultant/staff on call.

Medical record chart (patient file)

a) Trainees are expected to keep all charts current. All admission data (patient histories, physical and neurological exams), operative notes of trainee's cases[d], discharge summaries as well as consultation notes must be dictated or written down without delay. A daily progress note must be entered in the chart. Additional entries are required in case of particular events. Document the findings of all urgent diagnostic studies, especially MRT, CT, angiography immediately on the chart!

b) Postoperative orders and notes: At the end of surgery the trainee must write all orders for the ward/ICU on the respective order sheet, in particular arterial pressure and other limits, directives with regard to drains, positioning and mobilization, infusions and medications, and control examinations such as x-rays, MRI etc. It is expected that the trainee writes a short postoperative note in the chart regarding the result of surgery.

c) On Fridays, please document a neurological exam and outline a week-end plan! This will help the weekend trainees on call. Document all entries and orders on the chart with date, time and your name! Remember to order the drugs patients come with as well as drug levels (phenytoin, valproate, etc.). Address and inform the nurses also directly! This will help the nurses.

Responsibilities on wards and emergency unit

a) OP preparation
The trainee is responsible that for surgical procedures of the next day, the complete patient chart including all pertinent neuroradiological material for the operation is available on the ward on the evening before the operation. He will check and complete preoperative orders.

b) Emergencies and on call duties
The trainee on call should not be assigned to the routine OP programme of this day, so that he is available any time for emergencies[e]. Night duty starts at (16^{00}) hrs and lasts until (08^{00}) hrs the following morning.

Accurate lists concerning patients with open problems must be passed on to the next trainee on call. The patient list must be updated throughout the night or weekend on call.

On weekends there may be sometimes a more junior or a senior trainee and tasks have to be specified accordingly. Emergencies are primarily seen and examined by the trainee on call. He informs the respective consultant/staff on call and all further decisions are made together.

Problems arising with patients on the ICU or on the ward will be evaluated first by the trainee on call who will then rectify the problem or contact the consultant/staff on call. In case of major patient problems the trainee has to contact the consultant/staff immediately.

Information of patients and their relatives

The personal guidance and care of our patients is most important. Examinations and procedures should be explained in detail to the patient. The surgery has to be fully explained to the patient minimally 24 hours before a planned operation (Germany!), if necessary by means of a form or a schematic drawing. Risks have to be discussed and consent to the operation has to be obtained in written form [6]. The patient and the doctor and, in case of a major operation, preferably

d Consultant and trainee must discuss who will take care of the operative note. In general trainees will dictate the note if they have performed the majority of the procedure and consultants/staff will take care of the operative note for complex cases.

e This rule depends on local situation. If a junior and a senior house officer are assigned to on call duty, one of them can be involved in elective surgery to a limited degree.

another witness have to sign the form. When complex surgery is imminent, it is recommended to inform the next of kin. For children both parents have to agree with the operation and have to give their written consent. Information is usually given by the operating surgeon (or an assigned trainee).

Since nowadays patients are often admitted the evening prior to the operation only, it is advisable to inform the patient and obtain his consent already before, for example in the outpatient clinic.

Patients should be informed in a sensitive and caring manner about their disease, especially in case of an unfavourable prognosis. It is advisable to first interview the relatives and discuss with them in how much detail the patient can and wants to be informed. Information on the phone should be given only in exceptional cases or to personally well known relatives.

Discharge Procedures

The discharge summary must be ready at the time of discharge and a copy should be given to the patient. The discharge summary should be addressed to the referring physician. Family doctor and other involved colleagues also receive a copy. The discharge summary must contain the relevant diagnoses, procedures performed and a summary of the hospital course and outcome. Medications at the time of discharge must be listed and weaning instructions, if applicable, must be detailed. A follow-up date and time in the outpatient clinic should be scheduled prior to discharge and be mentioned in the discharge summary.

Prescriptions for necessary medications are handed to the patient upon discharge. In case of evening or weekend discharge, a supply of necessary medication for 24 hours is given to the patient.

Available medical reports and data sheets are put into the medical record chart together with the discharge summary. The completed chart is given to the ward secretary for final coding and archiving.

Outpatient consultations

On-call duty schedule and plan

Weekend and holiday regulations for ward and ICU rounds

Weekend and holiday ward rounds by the house staff on call are at (08^{30}) hrs. A briefing between the trainee leaving duty and the trainee beginning work is necessary (see 1.g.). Rounds on ICU start at (09^{00}). Problems on the ward are discussed with the chief trainee or the staff member on back-up call.[f]

Education, research and absences

Conferences, teaching rounds and education

a) *Journal club* (conference room, Tuesday 16^{00} till 17^{00}) [1, 7, 9, 10]
A journal club will be held twice monthly. The sessions consist of either current articles or a group of articles dealing with a common theme. The journal club has the purpose to review and discuss selected articles from the recent literature. Each trainee should review and present at least two articles per year. Articles can be selected with either a staff member or with the chief resident. The trainee learns to present the essence or "take home message", respectively, of the article but he should also learn to critically analyse whether the topic has been approached appropriately, whether methods applied are adequate, whether conclusions drawn from the results are balanced and not over- or under-estimated, and also whether they fit into the pertinent literature. Such a systematic approach is important for a trainee so that he acquires the ability to weigh the literature critically for its relation to his practice in neurosurgery.
b) *Afternoon teaching conference* (conference room, Tuesday 16^{00} till 17^{00} alternating with journal club)
Afternoon teaching rounds are mandatory and shall be attended by all trainees, students, and fellows unless they are in the OR.
c) *Weekly clinical neurosurgery conference (CNC)* (conference room, Friday 08^{15} till 10^{00})[g]
The CNC is dedicated to neurosurgical topics pertinent to the clinical service. All trainees, students, and fellows are expected to attend and to participate actively in this conference.

[f] Weekend procedures depend very much on local circumstances. A formal in-house briefing with the consultant/staff appears advisable if junior trainees are on call without back-up of a senior trainee.

[g] The classical grand rounds conference can be modified in many directions according to local circumstances. The here cited Friday morning model may not be appropriate in hospitals where Friday afternoon is already considered as part of the weekend. Upcoming working hour's regulations will also have a major impact on this traditional common teaching event.

d) *Monthly morbidity & mortality conference (MMC) [2, 3]* (conference room, Friday 08^{15} till 10^{00} instead of CNC)
The MMC reviews all mortalities, morbidities and complications of the service. The cases are selected by the consultant/staff and the trainees present the case. The consultant or trainee review the pertinent recent literature. The purpose of the MMC is future avoidance of occurred complications.

Presentations and Publications

Trainees should be well supervised during clinical and/or experimental research. They have to acquire skills to study and judge clinical case material. The following is a recommendation for presentations and publications

Y1: at least one poster presentation at a national congress/meeting
Y2+3: at least one poster and one oral presentation at a national congress or meeting
Y4–6: at least one poster and one oral presentation as well as one paper sent to a national or international journal for publication.

If a trainee presents a paper, poster or abstract at a meeting, expenses are/can be paid by the department according to prior individual agreement with the programme director.

Travel to meetings and courses

Trainees are encouraged to participate in meetings of the national society, meetings with special topics, or a neurosurgical course (European or national) and during year 4–6 also in some international meetings. Travel to meetings needs approval of the programme director and hospital administration. A travel request must be made at least 2 weeks prior to departure. Travel expenses are generally reimbursed if the resident contributes actively to the meeting. Financial support for courses is given according to prior individual agreement with the chairman.

Research leave

Concentrated periods of research in the lab or at another institution are encouraged and supported for trainees during the second half of training. The periods should range from 3 to 4 weeks and are generally allowed once or twice per year.[h] A fully detailed research project is a necessary condition. Co-ordination of the absence follows the procedures for vacations.

[h] Other models are a research rotation of 6–12 month's.

Vacation plan

Planned vacations must be permitted by the designated coordinator. Requests must be filed generally as early as possible. Requests will be generally accepted if at least 1 senior and 1 junior trainee remain on the respective ward during the absence. Replacement for other special duties, such as outpatient clinics and scheduled participation in conferences must be arranged by the trainee seeking leave of absence. No vacations are generally permitted during the national neurosurgical meeting.

Special management guidelines (standards of care, optional)

Guidelines for the management of all diseases are increasingly published by national and international organisations of medical specialists [12]. These guidelines focus usually on the available evidence and are rarely detailed enough to guide a resident. If standards of care are written for the department, the pertinent guidelines need to be concretised according to the tradition of the hospital. The authors have published such a manual in the German language [13].

Final remarks

These internal regulations have been designed with the intention to clearly define the duties and competencies of the trainees in order to avoid misunderstandings and mistakes as much as possible and to ascertain optimal patient management. They are not meant to be a rigid scheme for each single case. Initiative of one's own should be developed and be guided by personal conscience and knowledge.
Signature: Programme Director

References

1. Alguire PC (1998) A review of journal clubs in postgraduate medical education. J Gen Intern Med 13: 347–353
2. Bonsanto MM, Hamer J, Tronnier V, Kunze S (2001) A complication conference for internal quality control at the Neurosurgical Department of the University of Heidelberg. Acta Neurochir (Wien) [Suppl] 78: 139–145

3. Brennum J, Gjerris F Morbidity and mortality conferences. How we do it? This volume
4. Durning SJ, Sweet JM, Cation LJ (2003) Morning report: an analysis of curricular content and comparison to national guidelines. Teach Learn Med 15: 40–44
5. Li J, Tabor R, Martinez M (2000) Survey of moonlighting practices and work requirements of emergency medicine residents. Am J Emerg Med 18: 147–151
6. McClean KL, Card SE (2004) Informed consent skills in internal medicine residency: how are residents taught, and what do they learn? Acad Med 79: 128–133
7. McLeod PJ (1986) A successful formula for ward rounds. Cmaj 134: 902–904
8. Moberg-Wolff EA, Kosasih JB (1995) Journal clubs. Prevalence, format, and efficacy in PM&R. Am J Phys Med Rehab 74: 224–229
9. Pathak A, Pathak N, VKak K (2000) Ideal ward round making in neurosurgical practice. Neurol India 48: 216–222
10. Seelig CB (1991) Affecting residents' literature reading attitudes, behaviors, and knowledge through a journal club intervention. J Gen Intern Med 6: 330–334
11. Seelig CB (1993) Quantitating qualitative issues in residency training: development and testing of a scaled program evaluation questionnaire. J Gen Intern Med 8: 610–613
12. Steiger HJ (2001) Standards of neurosurgical procedures. Acta Neurochir (Wien) [Suppl] 78: 89–92
13. Steiger HJ (1999) (ed) Manual Neurochirurgie. Ecomed-Verlag, Landsberg

Correspondence: Prof. Dr. H.-J. Reulen, Schwojerstr. 19, 81249 Munich, Germany. e-mail: Ilona. Anders@med.uni-muenchen.de

Acta Neurochir (2004) [Suppl] 90: 39–50

Printed in Austria

VI Principles of teaching in a structured training programme, the rotations, and the surgical training plan

H.-J. Steiger

Department of Neurosurgery, Heinrich-Heine-University, Düsseldorf, Germany

Summary

The present paper is divided into two parts. In the first part it summarises *the essentials* of transfer of knowledge and personality from trainer to trainee. The training capacity of a programme should be identified first since the number of residents in training has implications on the structure of the programme. The capacity is limited by the number of surgical "resident cases", which should at least amount to 70 per year and resident. For the future, more emphasis should be laid on the acquirement of methods of self-teaching and continuous self-education, in order to provide the trainees with the ability to cope with changes during their later career more easily. In part two the organisation of rotations as well as the structured surgical training plan are discussed. Teaching can be organised either as a gradual exposure to more and more complex procedures or as a sequence of speciality rotations. Structured teaching of theoretical contents should accompany practical teaching and in academic programmes a scientific rotation should be integrated. The ongoing subspecialisation is currently exceeding the limits of complete coverage during a six-year-programme.

Keywords: Competence; neurosurgical residency programme; paedagogic principles; subspeciality training, structured curriculum, rotations, surgical training plan, self-directed learning.

Introduction

In a surgical speciality the transfer of practical skills in conjunction with the theoretical background allowing differential diagnosis and correct indication of procedures is of primordial importance. During the last decades, the number of procedures that need to be learned during residency training has steadily increased, and an unstructured programme cannot cover all necessary aspects within the available time. A sequence of well-defined clinical rotations with dedicated tutors is the simplest and most frequently used way and can presently be considered the standard way of achieving an efficient training. In these chapters the key aspects of organising such a training plan are dealt with. However, even with the advantages of a well-defined frame of rotations, it will not be possible anymore to accommodate up-coming new specialities within the available time. Therefore more flexible training plans shall be discussed, which can be implemented as alternatives to the standard system.

A. The transfer of knowledge and skills from trainer to trainee

Embedding of training in the hospital system

Training has always been an integral part of hospital life, but now the boundary conditions become more clearly defined in the context of hospital quality management programmes. As an example, the German KTQ® system (Kooperation für Transparenz und Qualität im Krankenhaus) shall be mentioned. In this system six *categories* are considered:

1. patient information
2. personnel management
3. hospital safety
4. data management
5. hospital planning
6. quality management

Category 2, personnel management, contains:

2.1. planning of personnel recruitment
2.2. personnel development
2.2.1. systematic concepts
2.2.2. definition of qualifications
2.2.3. training and education
2.2.4. financing of training and teaching
2.2.5. availability of training instruments
2.2.6. quality control of training

It is recommended that responsibilities of specific tasks are best delegated to the individual departments. The hospital or the university should provide the resources for the organisation of such tasks and the financing, respectively.

How many residents can be trained?

In general, comparing the number of resident cases can assess the training capacity of a unit and the required number of procedures required for board certification. If, for example, the national guidelines prescribe a number of 400 procedures done by each resident during a six-year programme, grossly 80 cases per year must be calculated for each resident in training. Depending on to which degree the staff members are committed to resident training, between 30 and 50% of all procedures can be resident cases (with a trainer supervising the procedure). Thus, there is a general recommendation that a total of about 250 cases will be needed per year to train one resident. If, for instance, a department has 1500 operations per year, between 5 and 6 residents can be trained at different levels. If the available number of resident cases is insufficient, it is better to limit the number of neurosurgical residents and fill the remaining assistant positions with rotating residents from other specialities.

The spectrum of cases in the training centre must also be considered. Although the total number of cases may be sufficient, deficiencies in specifically required areas of our speciality may limit the number of residents passing through the programme. If, for example, the number of cases in spinal surgery is very small at a university hospital specialised in complex intracranial surgery, the spinal sector limits the number of residents unless a training alliance is formed with a spinal centre, allowing the residents to spend a rotation in this unit.

The board certification requirements in most countries specify besides surgical experience, additional general and diagnostic experience, such as treatment plans, electrophysiological, ultrasound and radiological examinations, intensive care procedures and writing reports and expertises. Under most local circumstances, these aspects do not limit the training capacity, but may do so in special situations.

Numerical relations of trainer to trainees and who is teaching whom?

In the surgical disciplines learning by supervised doing is still prevailing due to the lack of surgical simulators or alternative methods for the transfer of surgical skills. Competence is measured in terms of experience. The ancient master-apprentice relation is still the key of surgical training.

Certain consideration must be given to the numerical relations between trainers and trainees. During a surgical procedure, practical knowledge can be transferred only to one resident while more theoretical knowledge can be transferred to small groups, for example during the planning conference for next day's procedures. In programmes with a well-defined rotation plan, a one-to-one relation (the tandem model) is ideal from the training point of view and ensures intensive transfer of practical and theoretical skills. If the trainee spends the day with one trainer, he participates intensively in patient care, decision making, planning of procedures, reflections concerning risks, the operation, the postoperative care and the follow-up.

In the one-to-one-system, the consultant primarily teaches the basic procedures and the openings. In a one-to-one system usually only one house staff is available for night on-call duty and the consultant needs to come in for surgical procedures. This close relationship ensures that procedures are learned in a specific manner according to the general agreements of the attending staff-group. Since learning surgical skills during a residency programme fills only part of the daily activities, it also appears conceivable that one trainer serves two residents (double-tandem model), a senior and a junior resident. The senior resident is directly engaged in the more complex cases and also can supervise the junior resident in the so-called component parts of the operation, for example the opening and closure. From the training point of view this may be less ideal, but two residents per trainer accommodates well the realities and necessities of hospital life.

As indicated, the one staff per two residents principle works well for neurosurgery. This principle allows also that the senior resident is involved in training the junior resident. During elective cases the senior resident will instruct the junior resident how to perform the opening or parts of the procedure, and if the on-call service is provided by a team of two, also the senior resident will teach the junior in the area of emergency procedures during the night, provided the local legal regulations allow such a system. If this principle is accepted for the training programme, one must be aware that the style of the basic procedures evades to a large degree the influence of the attending staff. The style of craniotomies is transferred from one senior resident generation to the next. Corrective influence from the staff becomes apparent only in the course of working up complications. The positive aspect of this system is that all three participants benefit. For the junior resident the effect is the same, whether instructed by the senior resident or by attending staff, the senior resident can develop teaching skills and the attending staff gets some time off for other duties.

The total number of trainers/consultants and residents certainly is influenced by a number of factors, i.e. size of department, number of procedures, presence of subspecialties, academic involvement, etc. In programmes with a large case load usually a relation of one to one is given but in some smaller programmes residents may represent under the present conditions a minority.

Up-coming legal regulations with the new European working hours legislation, especially "off" time after on-call duty, in the future will have an increasing and severe impact on the organisation of training. The requirement to go home after a night on call or to have some days off following a weekend on call, prolongs the necessary time span to obtain the required numbers of procedures performed and disturbs the rotations. Eventually it may lead to prolongation of the presently obligatory 6 years of training. A major additional effect is the uncoupling of the teacher/trainee relation if the trainee cannot spend anymore his whole time with his trainer. There is no question that training is less intensive or effective if the resident works with different trainers at the same time. Although there is presently not enough experience of how the training can be organised under such aggravated circumstances, the double tandem model may offer some advantages. On-call duties or time off respectively may be organised in a way that always two of the trio are working together, thus maintaining the necessary continuity for the physicians as well as the patients.

Written contents of training rotations and learning objectives

The aims and the contents of the individual rotations including theoretical knowledge and the type and number of diagnostic and operative procedures should be available in written form. This is important to frame the expectation of the trainee and to guide the teacher as well. Furthermore only written curricula allow internal or external quality control of the programme and only written learning objectives allow assessment of the trainee. An example of the curriculum for the rotation "Stereotactic and functional neurosurgery" could look as described in appendix 1.

When such curricula are developed, there is a trend for inclusion of everything in the speciality. It must be accepted that at the more junior or middle level the procedures to be performed cannot exceed the simple routine procedures. The subspeciality rotation shall create a platform for the trainee allowing for self-development thereafter.

Balance of theoretical and practical teaching

Although practical skills are of overwhelming importance in a surgical discipline, the theoretical background and knowledge should not be neglected and also be offered in a structured fashion. This is particularly important since the resident cannot autonomously recognise the importance of theoretical knowledge, and the programme director and the teaching staff must foster this notion systematically. In today's evidence driven medical world only knowledge of the pertinent literature allows for critical and sound settling of surgical indications. Theoretical knowledge needs to be subdivided into textbook material and recent literature. Besides recommending specific textbooks, the textbook material can be periodically covered in a dedicated conference.

However, this usually exceeds the local potential. A more effective way is to encourage trainees to participate in either the European training courses or comparable national courses, which cover most of the relevant areas in 4 or 5 dedicated courses. The residents must also be assisted with the acquisition of recent material. A "Journal Club" is a time proved forum to point at important new papers and to sharpen critical reading of scientific papers. The residents should also be encouraged to read the important neurosurgical journals. The increasing number of journals renders a clear recommendation unavoidable with regard to the expected reading. It is realistic for residents to read 2 or 3 core journals. A debatable question is whether the residents should be incited to read the journals already at the beginning of the residency or only later. Only if they begin reading early, they will survey the relevant literature at the end of their training. They will be able to discuss with experts at that point and they will be accepted. It is one of the important (but also difficult) duties of the Programme Director and the attending staff to create an educational environment with discussions on approaches, etc: readiness to learn new facts, methods and techniques becomes an integral part of clinical life.

It is an illusion to expect that anybody is able to survey the vast amount of new and potentially important publications in all the subspecialities of our field. The horizon can be somewhat enlarged beyond the core journals if a culture of communication with the subspecialists is encouraged. If, for example, the neuro-oncologist tracks a potentially important paper in a subspeciality journal, he should discuss this with the residents either on rounds or in the journal club. As soon as such a culture is established, it will be beneficial for all sides, and also the consultants will begin to learn from information coming from the residents.

External courses

Some important practical concepts cannot be conveyed locally without inadequate efforts. Trainees should be supported to attend specific hands-on training courses of their respective level of training. Examples are the following:

- microvascular anastomosis course
- anatomical dissection courses
- hands-on courses on specific approaches and techniques
- rhetoric courses, etc.

B. The rotations and the surgical training plan

According to the European Training Charter a department has to develop a Rotation Plan describing the training periods during the 6 years of training. Rotations in general are of 6 months' duration although some may be shorter. The idea is to structure these 6 years and not leave them at random. It is recognised today that covering all main areas of our speciality and teaching the many procedures is only possible within the frame of a strict organisation. For some departments it will be necessary to organise specific training periods in another neurosurgical unit, if adequate exposure in one area cannot be provided. It is also important to keep in mind that the allocation of rotations should preferentially be governed by the requirements of the training programme and not mainly by the needs of work on the wards! Experience from many institutions teaches that often conflicts may arise between the interests of clinical work and maintenance of the rotation schedule.

When planning a rotation schedule it should primarily be defined how much time shall be spent with non-neurosurgical activities (neurology, surgical disciplines, neuropathology, neuroradiology, research, etc.). The mandatory 48 months to be spent with clinical neurosurgery are an absolute minimum to teach the full variety of modern neurosurgery. In order to ascertain that all trainees have the same exposure, a rigid sequence of rotations is preferable. This allows an objective assessment and comparison of trainees' progress after each of the rotation periods.

A rotation plan can be developed in increasing order of comprehensiveness according to local possibilities and facts. A few examples shall be given.

The traditional model

In the traditional model that is dominated by generalist neurosurgeons, residents are involved in all cases on a ward and thus see always the broad spectrum of the speciality. They gradually grow into more responsibility according to the curriculum of the department.

It is recommended to assign trainees to a certain trainer during each rotation. This is more effective than working together with several staff members of whom no one has any defined responsibility. It also avoids the widely known problem where trainers give preference to active trainees and try to work together

Table 1. *Example A: the traditional model*

	Period 1	Period 2
Year 1	neurology or surgical discipline	neuropathol./ neuroradiology
Year 2	NS (Ward A)	NS (Ward B)
Year 3	intensive care	NS (Ward C)
Year 4	paediatrics (outside)	research
Year 5	NS (ward A)	NS (Ward B)
Year 6	NS (ward C)	subspeciality interest
Year 7	instructor, subspeciality interest or change to other department	

Example A is often used in smaller departments with 2–4 neurosurgical trainees and generalist neurosurgeons as trainers. In this example there are 2 or 3 wards. Trainee spends 6 months in intensive care and spends a 6 months' rotation in paediatrics (or any other missing area) in another unit outside. The last rotation is spent in one of the subspeciality areas of personal interest. In this model, residents of different stages manage patient care on the ward together. Allocation to surgical procedures is usually done by a staff member.

with them as long as possible, which may leave the trainee with deficiencies in other areas. During an assignment period (rotation) the trainer should have a clear responsibility to instruct and supervise a trainee to perform the procedures of the respective level (of the surgical training plan).

In this example it is further recommended to assign certain operative procedures, activities, and teaching to each one of the rotations. A structured surgical training plan allows for a continuous and systematic escalation of surgical responsibilities and competence through training years 1–6. A typical and widely used plan is presented in Appendix 2. Required minimum and/or average operative case numbers for each category can be assigned for each training year. A trainee is expected to fulfil the minimum numbers listed for the respective training period. This allows to detect deficiencies very early and correct them.

The subspecialist oriented rotation plan

In a department where several subspecialists are present, residents can work together with the consultants in specific subspeciality rotations. Training is provided through successive subspecialities according to a rotation schedule. The subspecialist groups can be organised with one staff and one or two residents or a fellow, respectively. If a department has a particular focus, e.g. functional or vascular neurosurgery, more than one staff member may share the workload in these subspecialities (Table 2).

Table 2. *Example B: subspeciality oriented rotation plan*

	Period 1	Period 2
Year 1	neuroradiology/ICU and neurotraumatology	neurology or surgical speciality
Year 2	functional and stereotactic NS, pain	neuro-oncology and neuropathology
Year 3	spinal NS	paediatric NS, epilepsy surgery
Year 4	research	research
Year 5	skull base and pituitary or spine and peripheral nerves	vascular NS
Year 6	neuro-oncology	free for subspeciality interest
Year 7	instructor or subspeciality interest, or change to other department	

In this example the trainee has rotations in all areas of neurosurgery. During neurotraumatology he is assigned to ICU, during neuro-oncology he has exposure to neuropathology, etc. Allocations to surgical procedures are done by his trainers. This is an example and can be changed in any way.

In this system it is necessary that all staff members and residents provide basic care and general neurosurgery. In practice a call schedule consisting of a staff person and one or several residents covers traumatology and other emergencies. In addition all staff members and residents care for elective cases not assigned to a specific subspeciality. This general root is a slim variant of the generalist-dominated programme. Knowledge and skills in the general aspects are also acquired over the years of training in a stepwise fashion. An example of a surgical training plan is presented in Appendix 3.

The subspeciality-dominated rotations have some advantages. The concentration on one subspeciality allows to see and perform more of the same procedures in a row (repetition effect) and focuses reading and acquisition of theoretical knowledge. Working with a competent subspecialist provides a deep and comprehensive insight and also renders account of the increasingly complex field of neurosurgery.

The limited time in the rotations certainly is not sufficient for a resident to acquire a level of expertise in the respective area. However, the resident is able to select one of these subspecialties for an additional fellowship. If neurosurgery shall survive in the border areas to other disciplines, such as carotid surgery or spinal instrumentation, specific subspeciality training is unavoidable.

Organisation of the rotation schedule in this example on the other side is not without problems. One question that needs to be solved with the staff members is how the sequence of rotations shall be established. It certainly would be problematic if a resident were exposed to clip an aneurysm during the first year of training. In general, all subspecialists argue that their discipline be reserved to the last two years.

Another problem is how many subspecialities can be accommodated in the six years of training. If all possible areas are included as six-month-rotations, and if a scientific year is integrated, the available time will be exceeded. We have made the experience that some rotations which are not too busy can be combined, which means that one resident works together with two staff members. When planning the rotation schedule, it is conceivable to divide the subspecialities into mandatory and optional rotations. The optional rotations should be done at the end of training in order to preclude premature commitment. A model could be to organise the four mandatory clinical years in a standard manner, have one year free for research or

Table 3. *Example C: variable subspeciality oriented program*

Subject	Total months (weeks)	Year of training					
		I	II	III	IV	V	VI
General surgery or traumatology							
Neurology							
Neurophysiology							
Neurotraumatology							
Neuroradiology							
Microsurgery (course)							
Neuropathology							
Spinal neurosurgery I							
Spinal neurosurgery II							
Peripheral nerves							
Rehabilitation							
Stereotactic and functional, pain							
Epilepsy surgery							
Intensive care							
Neuro-oncology							
Paediatric neurosurgery							
Vascular neurosurgery							
Research							
Skull base and pituitary							
Hands-on courses							
European or national training courses							
Medical laws							
Hospital economics							
No of months							
No of examinations							

In this example the various possible rotations and courses are listed (and can be completed), the total time in months or weeks is determined and finally the rotations and courses are assigned to the year of training. This example allows organising a core training programme of the 4 mandatory clinical years and then an individual shaping of the residual time. Instead of performing neurology or research, a second rotation in spinal neurosurgery can be chosen.

other commitments, and have 6–12 months as flexible rotations.

A variant of a subspeciality oriented rotation schedule is presented in Example C.

Rigid or flexible rotations?

The goal of a training programme is to assure that residents completing training have achieved the highest possible level of competency. The easiest way to ascertain that all residents have the same chance to reach this ideal is to define a rigid sequence of rotations such as in the previous example. All residents pass through all rotations.

In addition, the rigid schedule is the most simple and practical model to organise. The introduction at our institution proved to be a big step ahead with regard to resident competency at each level, particularly at the end of training. There was a constantly growing acceptance of responsibility and of independence. Also some aspects of competency-based training [4] can be included, thus allowing a certain amount of flexibility. Talented residents in each rotation could do numerically more operations as well as advance faster to complex procedures without disturbing the whole programme. This kind of flexibility exists in fact in most institutions.

A more *flexible curriculum* is certainly conceivable, particularly toward the end when, for instance, the last year can be tailored to the individual trainee's interest. The last year may be used either as an intensified academic training with research, as a rather practical training for residents aiming at private practice, or as a preparation for a subspeciality fellowship. A separation between academic neurosurgery and non-academic neurosurgery at an early stage is not desirable. On the other side, even academic programmes should not consider their research rotations mandatory but offer a more clinically oriented alternative for residents not interested in basic research [3]. Moreover, crossover should be accepted and structurally included. If a resident does not succeed in basic or clinical research or realises that he does not enjoy lab work, a crossover to a purely clinical curriculum should be welcome.

D. Long proposed a flexible way through the stages of residency according to competency [4]. In his competency based training scheme a talented resident could advance much faster to complex procedures than less gifted colleagues. From the theoretical point of view the competency-based scheme is convincing. There is little doubt, however, that organising a competency-based programme represents a considerable challenge for the programme director. It can happen that two or more residents end up at the same level simultaneously, which can exceed the case resources of a training programme. Collisions are certainly less likely if the number of residents is small in comparison with the number of staff.

Assessment of rotations

At the end of each training period or rotation an assessment of the trainees' progress is obligatory and performed by the supervising consultant [6]. The most practical way to assess surgical progress is the Logbook, the general progress of knowledge and skills by using an Evaluation Form. Details of the proceedings are described in the respective chapters. The assessment process allows not only an assessment of the trainee but also of the responsible tutor, and therefore is an instrument for programme optimisation.

In a teaching programme with a distinct junior (first 2 or 3 years) and senior level with different responsibilities, it may be appropriate or desirable to make an additional assessment prior to entering the senior resident level. Such midterm evaluation should include the following key points:

Midterm evaluation

Knowledge
- familiarity with the management standards of the service [9]
- text book material

Practical skills
- competence with lumbar discectomy and laminectomies
- competence with external cervical stabilisation (Halo etc.)
- competence with ventriculostomies and ventricular shunts
- competence with craniotomies
- competence with evacuation of intracranial haematomas

Scientific assessment (optional)
- publications
- actual projects

In order to prevent failure at the board exams and also to be able to guarantee for the performance of the residents released into independent practice, some departments organise an internal practical exam where residents have to demonstrate their competence in some procedures including the preparation and postoperative care of these patients. Assessment of theoretical knowledge in an objective and reproducible way is not possible for the individual training programmes and therefore programmes increasingly recommend their trainees to participate in the EANS written examination (see specific chapter).

Ways to go

The steadily growing amount of knowledge that needs to be acquired during residency training requires in each training centre the development of a well-structured written training curriculum. However, the old fashioned apprentice and master relationship remains the most important part of residency training, particularly in the subspeciality rotations, where the trainee collaborates with a specific tutor very intensely for a period of several months. During these rotations a major part of the knowledge and practical skills, and maybe also a portion of the personality of the specific tutor, is adopted. The responsibility of the trainer during these rotations cannot be overemphasised. The trainer cannot teach something different from what he is doing himself. To talk with Rudolf Steiner: the teacher must be a personification of the good, the true, and the beautiful. The child will accept what he really is and what he says [10].

In neurosurgery learning by doing still dominates despite efforts to develop simulators as used in aviation. The number of procedures performed as documented in the logbook is still the best way to estimate competence. In contrast, a pilot can be fully trained in a simulator and fly the real plane competently already at the first time. The availability of comparable neurosurgical simulators would allow a major step ahead in residency training. The crude "virtual manipulators" available today, however are rather toys than effective instruments. The reason for the insufficiency of "surgical trainers" appears not to be a principal one but a question of financial resources. In some surgical fields more progress has been made as compared to neurosurgery [8], and some specialities like anaesthesiology are easier objects for simulation [7]. Design and construction of a common platform of a surgical simulator allowing specification for the surgical specialities could be an affordable strategy for a company in the near future.

There are some principal questions with regard to the aims and methods of residency training. Major emphasis is currently put on conveying knowledge and skills. The fact that most knowledge and skills in medicine is relatively short-lived is not adequately accounted for. Many staff physicians stick for their entire career to what they have learned during residency. If certain methods become outdated, they just give them up without acquiring new ones. Therefore more weight should be put during residency on techniques of self-teaching and self-development. The paedagogic problems of self-directed learning are not trivial and are widely ignored in current continuous medical education (CME) programmes. One aspect is an intrinsic resistance to adult self-education. Hiemstra gives some practical hints with regard to overcoming this problem [2]. For learners, there are at least two factors that can be linked with resistance: self-concept and self-awareness. Many adults enter a teaching/learning transaction with low confidence and poor self-concept, making it initially difficult to take a high degree of responsibility for one's learning. Other learners, perhaps because of previous experiences with education, are simply not aware of the power they possess as learners and thus make the assumption that a highly teacher-directed approach is the way education "should" happen. Some of the strategies to address this concern include: self-reflection; peer reflection/judgements; interviewing techniques that allow individuals to learn from one another; generating lists of possible learning resources; portfolio review and assessment; journal writing; proactive reading; discussions (sharing with colleagues/peers); using learning contracts; and obtaining feedback from many different sources. The teachers can encourage self-education by several methods:

- Teach learners how to be self-reflective.
- Develop recognition of rewards for self-directed learning.
- Provide guidelines for organising and conducting self-directed learning projects.
- Help learners develop skill in using technology.
- Use technology for advisement and learner feedback.
- Help learners learn how to investigate options, opportunities, and resources.
- Help learners learn how to match individual strengths with interests.
- Help learners develop education/learning plans.
- Help learners develop good technical learning skills.
- Help learners feel comfortable with new content.
- Help learners enhance their sense of personal learning competence.
- Help learners develop confidence and skill in taking control of elements of the teaching/learning transaction (for example, needs assessment, goal

setting, selection of content and process, and self-evaluation).
- Help learners create and control effective learning environments.

Adult self-education does not principally differ from learning during childhood. Already at the end of the 19th century, John Dewey expressed a number of paedagogic concepts that are still valid [1]. The arising interests should be watched and fostered, not be repressed. To repress interest is to substitute the adult for the child, and so to weaken intellectual curiosity and alertness, to suppress initiative, and to deaden interest. The interest is always the sign of some power below; the important thing is to discover this power. This concept is easily applicable to residency training.

Appendix 1

Example of a curriculum of a subspeciality training rotation. Contents of training rotation "stereotactic and functional neurosurgery"

a) *Procedures and number to be performed under supervision*
   - stereotactic biopsy 10
   - stereotactic drainage of intracranial cysts/abscesses/haemorrhage 3
   - radiosurgical planning 5
   - functional electrostimulation of the spinal cord 5
   - functional deep brain stimulation 2
   - procedures for intrathecal morphine (baclofen) 5
   - Percutaneous selective trigeminal rhizotomy, or glycerol injection, respectively 5
   - microvascular decompression (Jannetta) 3

b) *Learning objectives [5]*
   - Choice of therapy for trigeminal neuralgia.
   - Indications and patient selection for spinal cord stimulation.
   - Benefits and disadvantages of infusion pumps.
   - Definition of factors guiding the choice of neuroimaging (CT, MRI, angiography) for stereotactic procedures.
   - The rationale for various MRI sequences used for tumour localisation and functional procedures.
   - The benefits and limitations of frame-based stereotactic procedures.
   - Patient selection for VL thalamotomy and pallidotomy and stimulation.
   - Advantages and disadvantages of ablative procedures.
   - Technical considerations to minimise the potential for an intracranial haemorrhage after a stereotactic biopsy.
   - Technical considerations to maximise the potential of diagnostic stereotactic biopsy.
   - Trajectories to biopsy a lesion in the pineal region, midbrain, pons, and medulla.
   - Advantages and disadvantages of radiosurgery and surgical resection for tumours and vascular malformations.

Appendix 2

Example of a surgical training plan

Year	Mandatory procedures*	Conditional procedures*
1	– spinal and ventricular taps, wound care – assistance at craniotomies – burr holes – opening and closing of procedures – nerve and muscle biopsies	– nerve decompression – lumbar discectomy – simple craniotomies – HALO
2	– elective convexity craniotomy – evacuation of epi- and subdural haematomas – cranioplasty – lumbar discectomy – impression fractures	– carpal and ulnar tunnel decompression – ventricular shunts
3	– posterior fossa and skull base craniotomies – lumbar and thoracic laminotomies – intracerebral haematomas – superficial meningiomas and gliomas – ventricular shunts – more complex traumatology (simple basal CSF leak) – spinal metastasis	– cerebellar haematoma – ventral approach to cervical spine – cervical laminotomies
4	– cerebellar haematomas – ventral and dorsal approach to cervical spine – spinal stenosis – cerebral metastases	– cervical discectomy – extraforaminal lumbar discectomy
5	– extraforaminal lumbar discectomy – cervical discectomy – intradural extramedullarytumours	– cervical fusion with plates – peripheral nerve grafts
6	– posterior fossa tumours – skull base meningioma – peripheral nerve grafts – spinal instrumentation	– aneurysm clipping – transsphenoidal procedures – stereotactic operations

* It is important to emphasise that in this scheme the exposure to the mentioned problems and procedures is not limited to the year of primary exposure but that the experience in these areas is gradually expanded during the subsequent years. Required minimum or average operative case numbers for each category can be assigned for each training year. Any change in the sequence of procedures is possible. This is an example.

Appendix 3

Example of a subspeciality oriented surgical training plan

Year	General procedures[1)]	Speciality procedures[2)]
1	– spinal and ventricular taps, wound care – assistance at craniotomies – burr holes – opening and closing of superficial procedures – nerve and muscle biopsies	a) *ICU rotation* – invasive monitoring – intubation, ventilation
2	– elective convexity craniotomy – evacuation of epi- and subdural haematomas – trigeminal thermorhizotomies – cranioplasty – lumbar discectomy – impression fractures	b) *stereotactic & functional* – stereotactic biopsies – radiosurgical planning – microvascular decompression (Jannetta) c) *neuro-oncology + neuropathology* – removal of gliomas – craniotomies, posterior fossa craniotomies – removal of convexity meningiomas
3	– posterior fossa craniotomy – intracerebral haematomas – ventricular shunts – superficial brain tumours – laminotomy for spinal metastasis	d) *spinal rotation* – lumbar and thoracic laminotomies – ventral and dorsal approach to cervical spine – cervical discectomies – extraforaminal lumbar discectomy – cervical fusion with plates – spinal instrumentation e) *paediatric and epilepsy* – invasive monitoring – temporal resections – paediatric shunts – simple paediatric tumours
4	– cerebellar haematomas – spinal stenosis decompression – skull base craniotomies – cerebral metastases	
5	– extraforaminal lumbar discectomies – intradural extramedullary tumours	f) *pituitary & skull base rotation* – skull base craniotomies – more complex traumatology (simple basal CSF leak) – skull base tumours transsphenoidal procedures g) *neurovascular rotation* – aneurysm clipping – carotid endarterectomy – resection of cavernomas – EC-IC bypass
6	– posterior fossa tumours – peripheral nerve grafts	h) *neuro-oncology rotation (elective subspeciality interest)* – removal of gliomas, metastases, meningiomas, etc – craniotomy under local anaesthesia free for subspeciality interest

[1)] The exposure to the mentioned procedures is not limited to the year of first exposure, but experience in these areas is gradually expanded during the subsequent years.
[2)] In contrast in the subspeciality areas, exposure to the procedures is generally limited to the rotation. Any change in the sequence of procedures is possible. This is an example.

References

1. Dewey J (1897) My pedagogic creed. School 54: 77–80 (*http://www.pragmatism.org/genealogy/dewey/My_pedagogic_creed.htm*)
2. Hiemstra R, Brockett RG (eds) (1994) Overcoming resistance to self-direction in adult learning (No. 64) Jossey-Bass, San Francisco (*http://www-distance.syr.edu/learning.html*)
3. Kempski O (2001) Research and clinical routine in the next century: segregation or co-operative networks? Acta Neurochir (Wien) [Suppl] 78 : 213–216

4. Long DM (2001) Competency based residency training. The next advance in graduate medical education. Acta Neurochir (Wien) [Suppl] 78: 153–158
5. Neurosurgery://on-call (AANS-CNS website), professional pages, residency curriculum (*http://www.neurosurgery.org/resident/curriculum/index.html*)
6. Reulen HJ (2001) The semi-annual residency rotation summary: a means to assess the quality of neurosurgical training. Acta Neurochir (Wien) [Suppl] 78: 159–164
7. Schwid HA, Rooke GA, Carline J, Steadman RH, Murray WB, Olympio M, Tarver S, Steckner K, Wetstone S (2002) Evaluation of anesthesia residents using mannequin-based simulation: a multiinstitutional study. Anesthesiology 97: 1434–1444
8. Seymour NE, Gallagher AG, Roman SA, O'Brien MK, Bansal VK, Andersen DK, Satava RM (2002) Virtual reality training improves operating room performance: results of a randomized, double-blinded study. Ann Surg 236: 458–463
9. Steiger HJ, Reulen HJ (1999) Manual Neurochirurgie. Landsberg, Ecomed-Verlag
10. Steiner R (1923) Die Erziehung des Kindes vom Gesichtspunkte der Geisteswissenschaft. Ein Vortrag über Pädagogik. Rudolf-Steiner-Verlag (edn 1992)

Correspondences: H.-J. Steiger, M.D., Neurochirurgische Klinik, Universitätsklinikum, Moorenstraße 5, 40225-Düsseldorf, Germany. e-mail: Steiger@uni-duesseldorf.de

Acta Neurochir (2004) [Suppl] 90: 51–57

Printed in Austria

VII A structured neurosurgical training plan and the neurosurgical logbook in the UK

K. W. Lindsay

Department of Neurosurgery, Southern General Hospital, Glasgow, UK

Introduction

Although there are many similarities in neurosurgical training methods throughout Europe, some differences exist in training programmes and the extent of practical experience trainees gain in different countries.

In the UK a structured neurosurgical training plan and a log-book have a long tradition for over 20 years and are mandatory for any training programme. The UK training programme aims to produce a neurosurgeon capable of independent practice, wholly responsible for patients admitted under his/her care. This requirement perhaps differs from some other European countries where a hierarchical system exists and the newly trained neurosurgeon has limited autonomy. Whatever system is present, learning does not stop on gaining accreditation, but should persist throughout the neurosurgeon's entire working career.

A structured training plan should ensure that the trainee has gained adequate exposure to a wide variety of neurosurgical conditions in a training unit with appropriate facilities and has attended a weekly educational programme covering the necessary range of academic disciplines. It is essential that such a training programme be combined with a robust method of assessing progress. Ensuring that the trainee completes a specific number of years within a training programme is straightforward, but determining whether or not he/she has achieved the required level of knowledge and the required level of clinical and operative competence at each stage of training presents challenging difficulties.

To become competent in performing an operative technique begins with observation, followed by supervised guidance by a patient teacher. Finally experience by repetition improves ability, increases confidence and provides increasing exposure to anatomical variations and to potential complications. The maintenance of an operation logbook records such experience and is an important aspect of a structured training programme.

This chapter sets out guidelines to establish a comprehensive, structured and balanced neurosurgical training programme, based primarily on the system currently used in the United Kingdom and Ireland. It also describes the neurosurgical logbook and reviews the cumulative operative totals achieved by UK/Irish trainees over the last decade. The use of operative totals in assessing progress and attainment is reviewed along with other methods of determining competence in chapter XI on page 77. These continue to evolve in the need to maintain standards and to ensure that trainees achieve satisfactory training.

It is hoped that those countries in which training is less well structured may take up these suggestions and provide an opportunity to establish a more uniform approach to training throughout Europe according to the UEMS Training Charter, the respective recommendations of the UEMS Section of Neurosurgery and the Joint Residency Advisory and Accreditation Committee.

The structured training plan

Objectives

Neurosurgery is a specialty dealing with the diagnosis, evaluation and treatment of patients with disorders of the cranium, spine and nervous system. On completing training, the trainee must be capable of practising general neurosurgery competently and independently and should develop a special expertise in at least one of the subspecialties and/or research.

It is not expected that trainees on completion of training, should attain competence in every operative procedures (see Table chapter XI). When not competent to deal with all aspects of a particular condition, the trainee should have sufficient knowledge and expertise to care for such a patient until referral to an appropriate neurosurgeon is arranged.

Requirements for entry into neurosurgical training

Although such requirements will vary from country to country these should be clearly specified. It is suggested that trainees should not enter a neurosurgical training programme immediately after gaining a medical degree, but should obtain experience at a junior level in other surgical specialties as well as in neurosurgery. Such exposure may help convince a trainee that he/she has made the correct career choice before embarking on a prolonged period of training. During this time the trainee should acquire knowledge of the management of surgical patients in general e.g. – wound healing, fluid balance, coagulation and thrombotic disorders, pain control, triage, assessment and resuscitation after trauma, airway control, respiratory problems and ventilation, chest, abdominal and limb injuries, blood pressure control, sepsis and shock, multi-system failure, principles of oncology and the principles of outcome assessment after surgery.

In the UK such knowledge is tested by an MCQ, an oral and a clinical examination on basic surgical training. In addition trainees must attend and satisfactorily complete a five day course on basic surgical skills.

Recommendations

- Six months general surgery
- Six months orthopaedic surgery (including emergencies)
- Six months accident and emergency
- Six months neurosurgery

Duration of neurosurgical training in the UK

In most instances it is expected that neurosurgical training should last a *minimum of six years* consisting of

- *Five years in clinical neurosurgery* which must incorporate six months of *paediatric neurosurgery*. During this training period, the trainee must acquire a good working knowledge of neuroradiology, neuropathology and neurophysiology, although he/she need not have worked in these specialties.
- *One further year of training* should be completed in any related branch of the specialty, e.g.,
  - laboratory or clinical research,
  - subspecialisation,
  - training overseas,
  - up to 6 months in neurology, neuroradiology, neuropathology or neurophysiology (more than one could be taken).

Alternatively, the trainee could complete a further year of clinical neurosurgery within his training unit. The trainee need not take this year at the end of training, particularly if undertaking research. Some may wish to extend a period in research to two or three years to attain a higher degree.

Rotational programmes

Since it may not be possible to incorporate all training requirements within a single neurosurgical unit, it may be necessary to set up rotational programmes incorporating two, three or even four units through which the trainees would rotate for specific periods. Such rotational arrangements would be essential

- in units with no (or limited) paediatric neurosurgery.
- in small units with limited bed numbers where less than four specialists/consultant neurosurgeons practice
- in units without access to research facilities.

Content of training programme

Because hours available for training vary, the content is *not prescriptive* with respect to each individual year of training. General principles apply and include –

In the first 2 years, the trainee must become competent at history taking, neurological examination, assessment of clinical problems, non operative management, neurosurgical intensive care, interpretation of neuroradiological, neuropathological and other neuroscience investigations and the basics of operating, e.g., should be able to perform craniotomies, for cranial trauma and malignant tumours, shunting procedures, procedures for lumbar disc disease and cervical degenerative disease. Reading should include standard neurosurgical texts and the major neurosurgical journals.

In years 3 and 4 the range of conditions operated upon should widen to include benign tumours and posterior fossa procedures.

In years 5 and 6 the trainee should increase his/her experience of more major cases, e.g., benign tumours and aneurysms and develop some experience in more specialised fields, e.g., skull base surgery, transphenoidal pituitary surgery and pain.

Trainees especially during 5th and 6th years would be expected to be involved in the training of more junior neurosurgical trainees.

Neuroradiological, neuropathological and neurophysiological experience should be gained in relation to each clinical case, in addition to any coverage in the academic programme. Throughout the period of training, reading of journals should continue.

Research

All trainees are encouraged to undertake research and are expected to develop an understanding of research methodology during neurosurgical training. Up to one year of full-time research can count towards the six years of required neurosurgical training. Some trainees may wish to extend their period in research for a further year or two to obtain a higher degree. Research during the training programme should be supervised by a specifically named trainer with appropriate qualifications.

All trainees including those who do not undertake a specific piece of research will be expected to gain sufficient understanding of research and statistical techniques to permit assessment of published work.

Subspecialty training in neurosurgery

Trainees should be encouraged to develop a subspecialty interest provided this does not adversely affect training in general. The trainee may wish to spend up to one of the six years focusing on one or more subspecialty interests, e.g., skull base procedures, complex spinal procedures, functional neurosurgery, paediatric neurosurgery or complex vascular procedures. It is expected that most trainees would continue to develop a subspecialty interest beyond completion of their CCST.

Study leave

Trainees should have the opportunity to attend both national and international meetings in neurosurgery or in a neurosurgical subspecialty throughout their training. Trainees would be expected to attend at least one national neurosurgical society meeting per year. Where possible, expenses should be provided either wholly or partly to enable the trainee to attend. Trainees should also be encouraged to apply for EANS courses during the 2nd or 3nd year of training.

Training agreements

Some countries may require that a formal training agreement is drawn up between the body responsible for training and the trainee. This should define in terms of education and training, the relationship, duties and obligations on each side.

The training unit

It is expected that the facilities of any training unit would include

- at least 25 neurosurgical beds,
- either dedicated neurosurgical intensive care beds or access to intensive care beds within a general hospital,
- a 24 hour operating theatre with operating microscope,
- access to CT scanning and magnetic resonance imaging,
- access to other specialties including neurology, neurophysiology, neuroradiology, neuropathology, neuroanaesthesiology, neuro-otology, neuroophthalmology, maxillofacial surgery, general surgery, orthopaedic surgery, internal medicine,
- an accessible library with books and journals on neurosurgery,
- computer search facilities,
- an academic programme as specified below.

Academic programme (for UEMS-recommendations see p. 8, chapter I)

Each training unit should maintain an academic programme of neurosurgical/neuroscience education. This should be continuously available throughout the training period and should include

- Lectures, including visiting speakers and incorporating basic neurosciences
- Clinical presentations with all neuroscience disciplines
- Neuropathology including clinicopathological conferences
- Neuroradiological conferences
- Journal club
- Audit
- Research meetings.

Trainee assessment

No structured training programme is complete without a method of assessing trainee progress and attainment at regular intervals, followed by a final assessment leading to the award of the Certificate of Completion of Specialist Training (CCST). The methods currently used in the UK and Ireland are described in Chapter XI along with newer concepts for competence assessment.

Training programme assessment

In the UK, each training programme must be approved by the Specialist Advisory Committee (SAC) in Neurosurgery. This committee works on behalf of the Joint Committee for Higher Surgical Training (JCHST), supervising all surgical specialties for the four Surgical Royal Colleges, the bodies responsible for the standard of training. SAC members visit every training programme on a four-year basis to monitor standards and the quality of training in individual neurosurgical units. Both trainers and trainees are interviewed and facilities are inspected. The findings of the visit are documented in detail and reported to the whole SAC committee. The SAC decides on whether the volume of work is sufficient to provide adequate training material for the number of trainees in the unit and compares this with the actual experience gained. Such visits led to the withdrawal of recognition of training from six units over the last decade. All eventually regained recognition after introducing the recommended improvements.

The Joint Residency Advisory and Accreditation Committee (JRAAC), under the auspices of the UEMS and the EANS, now offer an equivalent accreditation facility for any European centre wishing to participate. Visits began in 2000. A number of centres from different countries have already taken up this offer.

The neurosurgical logbook

For over 20 years, trainees in the UK and Ireland have recorded operative procedures in which they have participated, either as assistant, or as the surgeon (with or without assistance) in a standardised logbook. From this they derive cumulative totals categorised under the headings listed in Table 1. These are reviewed by the Training Programme Director as part of the trainee's annual assessment. At the end of six years of training, each trainee submits his or her cumulative totals to the SAC as part of the accreditation process (see chapter XI).

The logbook categorises each procedure into the following groups:

P – The trainee has performed the operation. The consultant may have scrubbed to either see the pathology or because the trainee required an assistant, but the consultant must not have made a contribution/intervention significantly affecting the execution of the operation.

T – Trainee training a more junior trainee and assisting with the operation.

C – The trainee has done the operation with a consultant or a more senior trainee assisting or standing-by in the operating theatre and the supervisor making a significant decision or practical manoeuvre during the operation.

A – The trainee is the principal assistant at the operation.

Between 1990 and 2000, as both a member then chairman of the SAC in neurosurgery, I have compiled a database of operative totals for each trainee, permitting analysis of the range, mean and median totals for each procedure. For simplicity, any "T" procedure was reclassified as a "P".

Over the eleven year period, 109 trainees achieved accreditation or the CCST (introduced in 1996). Paediatric procedures were classified separately in 1997, increasing the operative categories from 50 to 74 (Table 1). Thirty-two trainees categorised paediatric procedures separately.

Operative totals

Table 1 shows the range and median values of operative totals over the decade for procedures carried out "personally" i.e. where the consultant may or may not be present, but if present, not making a contribu-

Table 1. *The median, mean and range of trainee operative totals performed 'personally' on completion of training**

Operative experience performed personally

Adults		Min	Max	Mean	Median
Head injuries	burr holes – ICP monitoring	0	131	35	32
	burr holes – ch. subdural	14	140	53	49
	craniotomy – extradural	8	60	25	23
	craniotomy – acute subdural	7	64	28	26
	craniotomy – intracerebral	2	37	12	9
	craniotomy – other	1	21	5	4
	depressed fractures	2	60	18	16
	dural repair	1	25	7	6
	combined craniofacial repair	1	28	4	3
	cranioplasty	0	46	11	9
Supratentorial tumours	biopsy	1	345	37	33
	stereotactic/Ids biopsy	0	142	28	23
	craniotomy – intrinsic tumour	11	162	52	49
	meningioma	8	38	18	17
	other benign	1	14	4	4
Midline tumours	transphenoidal	0	26	7	6
	other	0	9	2	1
Posterior fossa tumours	malignant	2	28	8	8
	acoustic	0	22	2	1
	other benign	1	33	7	6
Hydrocephalus	external ventricular drain	13	128	50	43
	shunts insertion	27	230	95	89
	shunt revision	5	171	43	35
	Arnold Chiari	1	11	4	4
Vascular	craniotomy – aneurysm	17	108	39	36
	craniotomy – AVM	0	11	3	3
	craniotomy – intracerebral haematoma	1	43	16	15
	posterior fossa haematoma	1	24	7	6
	craniotomy/craniectomy – other	0	3	1	1
	endovascular – aneurysm	0	0	0	0
	endovascular – AVM	0	0	0	0
	endovascular – tumour circulation	0	0	0	0
	carotid endarterectomy	0	26	2	0
Infection	abscess	2	66	11	10
	subdural empyema	0	14	5	4
	spinal abscess	0	8	3	3
Spine	cervical disc disease/spondylosis	21	149	59	54
	thoracic disc disease	0	11	1	0
	lumbar disc disease/spondylosis	5	343	101	88
	transoral	0	6	1	0
	syrinx	0	8	2	2
	dysraphism	0	8	2	1
	tumours – extradural	2	59	17	14
	tumours – intradural extramedullary	0	16	6	6
	tumours – intradural intramedullary	0	12	2	2
	spinal fixation	0	60	11	7
Pain:	trigeminal neuralgia – lesion	0	59	9	7
	trigeminal neuralgia – MVD	0	23	4	3
Functional	stereotaxy	0	46	3	0
	surgery for epilepsy	0	31	2	1

tion or intervention significantly affecting the execution of the operation. Inevitably numbers vary considerably depending on both the complexity of the procedure and its frequency of occurrence. For example, the highest median values exist for shunt insertion (89) and operations for lumbar disc disease (88). For relatively common but more complex procedures such as craniotomy for aneurysm repair and meningioma removal, trainees achieved median operative totals of 36 and 16 respectively. Few trainees performed per-

Table 1 (continued)

Operative experience performed personally					
Paediatric		Min	Max	Mean	Median
Head injuries	extradural	0	25	5	3
	other acute haematoma	0	12	3	3
	chronic subdural/hygroma	0	14	4	3
	depressed fracture	0	12	5	4
	ICP monitoring	0	80	16	12
Tumours	supratentorial	0	6	2	2
	infratentorial	0	9	3	2
	stereotactic/ids biopsy	0	16	3	2
Hydrocephalus	external ventricular drain	0	32	11	9
	shunt insertion	0	129	34	27
	shunt revision	0	102	29	26
	Arnold Chiari	0	2	1	0
	encephalocele	0	4	1	1
Spine	mening/meningomyelocele	0	70	3	1
	tethering syndromes	0	12	2	1
	tumours	0	5	1	1
Paediatric functional	spasticity	0	3	0	0
	surgery for epilepsy	0	5	1	0
Neuroendoscopy	adult	0	25	1	0
	paediatric	0	6	2	1
Craniostosis	sutural craniectomy	0	18	3	1
	combined craniofacial	0	4	1	1
Other	vascular	0	2	1	1
	infection	0	20	4	3

* From 1990 to 2000, 109 trainees were assessed. *ICP* Intracranial pressure; *AVM* Arteriovenous malformation; *MVD* Microvascular decompression.

sonally complex procedures such as for intradural intramedullary tumours or arteriovenous malformation, (median values of 2 and 3 respectively). No trainee performed unassisted a carotid endarterectomy, a thoracic disc removal or a transoral approach. A similar table was produced giving the range, mean and median totals for procedures carried out by the trainee, but assisted by the consultant, thus providing a guide to the extent of direct supervision.

It is important to note that the figures presented in Table 1 are the median totals actually achieved by trainees on completing their neurosurgical training. These reflect the service aspect of the training period as well as the training itself. They do *not* reflect the training committee's views of the minimum number required to achieve competence to perform a specific procedure. No one would claim that it is necessary to perform 89 adult shunt insertions to achieve competence for that specific procedure. No attempt has been made to define such numbers. Tables of operative totals were fed back to training programme directors from 1992 onwards. It was explained that the SAC expected trainee operative totals to 'approach the median value for the majority of procedures'.

Over the decade, no significant change occurred in the median number of operative procedures performed for each condition from one year to the next. Figure 1 indicates the median totals achieved each year for five

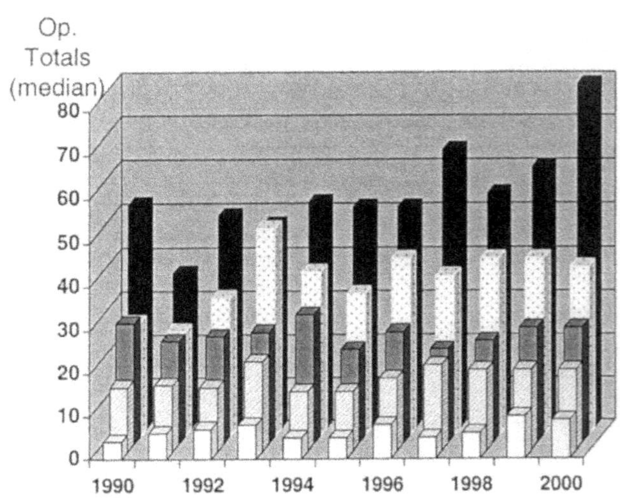

Fig. 1. The median operative totals achieved per year for five procedures from 1990–2000. The number of trainees achieving accreditation /CCST per year was respectively – 6, 12, 7, 5, 13, 14, 8, 9, 11, 13 and 11. ■ Cervical disc/spondylosis; ▨ Aneurysm; ■ Subdural; ▨ Meningioma; □ Transsphenoidal

key procedures. In particular, it is noted that the number of craniotomies for aneurysm and traumatic subdural haematoma remain constant despite the recent trend for coil embolisation and the reduction in trauma from road traffic accidents. With release of results from the ISAT trial (4), the number of patients undergoing direct aneurysm repair and subsequently the number of procedures performed by trainees will inevitably fall. In the future, trainees may only perform this procedure if they have expressed a subspecialty interest in vascular surgery.

Recording cumulative operative totals from the neurosurgical logbook provides an objective method of monitoring operative experience. To use this as a method of evaluating progress requires some caution. Although trainers check and countersign pages within the logbook, the categorisation of the procedure i.e., "P", "C", or "A" depends to some extent on the integrity of the trainee. Even with the best intentions, some variability must exist in deciding the extent of the trainers' participation. The "P" category has recently been sub-divided into "P = consultant available but not in the operating room" and "SU = consultant on standby in the operating theatre but unscrubbed". The "C" category has been redefined to mean, "surgeon scrubbed". These measures may help to reduce variability in recording the data and help identify the degree of supervision within theatre. Other pitfalls will be described in chapter XI.

References

1. Lindsay KW (2002) Neurosurgical training in the UK and Ireland: assessing progress and attainment. Neurosurgery 50: 1103–1113
2. Joint Committee on Higher Surgical Training (1996) A manual of higher surgical training in the United Kingdom and Ireland. Royal College of Surgeons of England London, (http://www.jchst.org/)
3. Joint Committee on Higher Surgical Training. (Supplement) (1996) A curriculum for higher training in neurosurgery. Royal College of Surgeons of England London (http://www.jchst.org/)
4. International Subarachnoid Aneurysm Trial (IASA) Collaborators Group (2002) Lancet 360: 1267–1274

Correspondence: K.W. Lindsay, Department of Neurosurgery, Southern General Hospital, Govan Road, Glasgow G51 4TF, UK. e-mail: kwlindsay@sgh.scot.nhs.uk

Acta Neurochir (2004) [Suppl] 90: 59–66

Printed in Austria

VIII The European Neurosurgical Log-Book (UEMS/EANS)

H.-J. Reulen

Department of Neurosurgery, Klinikum Großhadern, Ludwig-Maximilians-University, Munich, Germany

In the European Training Charter (1), Chapter 6, 1.B.1, the use of a log-book for neurosurgery is specified as mandatory: "The candidate neurosurgeon should keep an authorized log-book of operative experience". Chapter 5.3 formulates the requirements for trainees: "The trainee should keep his/her personal log-book or equivalent up-to-date according to national rules and EC directives as well as considering UEMS/European Board recommendations."

Written documentation of the operative procedures done by a resident and attested by the signature of the supervising trainer/programme chairman is presently required in more or less all European countries. A compilation in tabular form of all surgical procedures is also called for in the national board examination and the formal recognition as a specialist, respectively. However, the many European Neurosurgical Societies, as a consequence of their different historical background and development, employ a variety of systems and categories of procedures.

With growing consciousness for a uniform European Resident Training Programme of high standard, it became necessary to develop a modern edition of a Neurosurgical Log-book to allow for documentation of the broad variety of surgical procedures of today's neurosurgery with its various subspecialties.

The present Neurosurgical Log-Book was developed in 1997/98 by the Residency Advisory Committee of the EANS (later JRAAC), based on the long-term experience of our colleagues in the UK, the USA, and other national societies where such a system for documentation of surgical procedures is used regularly. Experienced individuals from many national societies have contributed to the new European log-book with their proposals and advice. The Log-Book has been approved by the Administration Council of the EANS (June 1998) and by the Section of Neurosurgery of the UEMS as the official European Log-Book in Neurosurgery.

In this European Log-book procedures have been included that are of relevance in a modern neurosurgical training programme. The log-book really represents the common European suggestion for a core education in our specialty. Thus trainees during their 6 years of training should be adequately exposed to the respective diseases and operative procedures, and they should demonstrate that they have acquired the necessary competency called for.

If a training site cannot offer exposure in one or more fields of our specialty, they must seek collaboration with another training site so that residents will also receive that missing part. In future two or even three training sites will have to organise one common training programme. This will require a certain degree of flexibility, but some countries have already demonstrated that it is possible.

Explanations how to use the Log-Book

The Neurosurgical Log-Book written in English is intended to be a record of all operations the trainee performs or participates in during his training. In consecutive order the date of operation, patient's name, and nature of the operation should be entered on the pages as indicated (Table 1). The last column of the page serves to designate the exact role of the trainee during the operation. Operations are to be classified into *one* of the four following groups. For the national or European Board examination, the two groups T and TS are to be considered when preparing the consolidated list of operation.

Table 1.

Date of operation	Patients number	Patients name	Nature of operation	S, TS, C, A

T The trainee has done the operation. The supervising consultant must not have made a decision/practical manœuvre during the operation.

TS The trainee has done the operation, but the supervising consultant has made a significant decision/practical manœuvre during the operation.

C The trainee has performed component parts during the operation under supervision of a senior surgeon: positioning, operative approach (i.e. craniotomy, opening, closure, drainage, draping, written instructions for postoperative care).

A The trainee is the principal assistant during the operation.

At the end of the log-book there is a consolidated list of all procedures which are of relevance in a modern training programme, divided into "adults" and "paediatrics" (Table 2).

Categorisation of groups T and TS depends to some extent on the integrity of the trainee. Even with the best intentions some variability will exist between trainees and centres. Also in some countries, legislation strictly requires trainees to be closely supervised during a procedure while in others it is sufficient for the trainer to be available but not necessarily present in the operation theatre. It is wise, therefore, to add T and TS groups when recording cumulative operative totals.

The log-book must be supervised and signed by the Programme Director or the responsible tutor at regular intervals.

The log-book can be conducted in form of a booklet and can be obtained free of charge through Aesculap AG + Co KG, P.O. Box 40, D – 78501 Tuttlingen (attn. Mrs. Eva Streit), who have generously financed the print. Recently an electronic version has been developed by the Joint Residency Advisory and Accreditation Committee with the financial support of the EANS. This electronic version can be downloaded from the EANS web site (*www.EANS.org*) and managed by oneself. The version is self-explanatory and leads the user in a simple and logic sequence through the programme. The booklet, and more easily the electronic version, allows to establish a consolidated list of operations performed during any desired period, for instance during a specific rotation, on an annual or semi-annual basis, or for the entire 6 years of training. It permits the trainer to assess a trainee's progress at regular intervals for evaluating a rotation and his growing autonomy. It also allows to detect any possible deficiencies in the operative training very early so that they can be corrected. Furthermore it permits to register components of an intervention and the degree to which the trainee has been involved. This offers the possibility to observe the progress of a trainee as well as his growing autonomy.

It allows also a comparison between different trainees as well as between different training centres. Finally it can be used, optionally or already obligatory as in some European countries, as the required documentation for national or European Board examinations.

In future this official European Neurosurgical Logbook will be requested for departments who wish to participate in the European Accreditation and Certification Process.

Conclusions

The introduction of a common European Log-book was certainly a big step forward in the endeavour to organise a well-structured European residency training programme. Its advantage is to have a clear and comparable system for documentation of all surgical interventions in which a trainee has been involved. It precisely fulfils the requirements of the European Training Charter. Following its introduction, several national societies and many departments have already made its use mandatory for their trainees, and in a not too distant future we hope that all member societies of the EC formally will have implemented this Log-book.

Some national societies may wish to use the Logbook in their own language. If the electronic version in a national language is desired, the JRAAC can help to supply this at a reasonable price.

In the previous chapter the experiences with a fairly similar log-book used in the United Kingdom and Ireland are presented, where a structured training programme has already been in existence for many years. In this article many interesting and essential data are reported which are of importance for everyone who is to organize or improve a training programme.

An important question is whether each trainee needs to be competent in all of the very complex procedures of the entire speciality. Must each one of the trainees have done a large amount of aneurysms, acoustic neurinomas or insertion of a fixateur in a traumatic lumbar spine fracture, to name some of the typical, complex interventions? It is recognised that our specialty has grown rapidly to a point where one individual probably no longer is in a position to cover all

Table 2. *Consolidated list of operations performed*

ADULT

	NATURE OF OPERATION	T	TS	C	A
1.	**Head Injuries**				
	Burr holes: ext. ventricular drainage/ICP-monitoring/reservoir				
	exploration/chronic subdural				
	Extradural haematoma				
	Acute subdural haematoma/contusion				
	Intracerebral haematoma				
	Depressed skull fracture				
	Gunshot / Penetrating wound				
	Dural repair (CSF fistula)				
	Combined craniofacial repair				
	Cranioplasty				
	Others				
2.	**Supratentorial Tumours and Lesions (excl. stereotactic procedure)**				
	Primary/intrinsic tumours				
	Metastatic lesions				
	Meningioma				
	Other benign lesions (Craniopharyngioma)				
	Pituitary - transphenoidal approach				
	Pituitary - transcranial approach				
	"Craniotomy Flap"				
	Others				
3.	**Posterior Fossa Lesions**				
	Primary and metastatic tumours				
	Acoustic neurinoma				
	Meningioma				
	Other benign lesions (abscess, epidermoid, etc.)				
	Arnold Chiari malformation				
	Others				
4.	**Infection**				
	Abscess				
	Subdural empyema				
	Others				

Table 2 (continued)

ADULT

	NATURE OF OPERATION		T	TS	C	A
5.	**Vascular**					
	Craniotomy:	Aneurysm				
		AVM				
		Intracerebral haematoma				
		Cavernous angioma				
	Endovascular:	Aneurysm				
		AVM				
		Tumour embolisation				
	Occlusive:	Bypass				
		Endarterectomy				
	Haematoma (spontaneous intracerebral)					
	Others					
6.	**Hydrocephalus** (≥16 years)					
	Shunting procedure, initial					
	Shunt-revision					
	Endoscopic fenestrations					
	External ventricular drainage					
7.	**Spine**					
	Cervical Disc Disease or Spondylosis					
		Anterior approach with (bone) graft				
		with (out) graft				
		with instrumentation				
		Posterior approach (foraminotomy)				
		with instrumentation				
		Laminotomy/Laminoplasty				
	Thoracic Disc Disease					
	Lumbar Disc Disease or Spondylosis					
		Lumbar disc				
		with instrumentation				
		Laminotomy/Laminectomy				
	Spinal Tumours					
		Extradural				
		Intradural: extramedullary				
		intramedullary				
		Instrumentation in vertebral tumours				
	Spinal Trauma					
		Decompression				
		Instrumentation				
	Others					

Table 2 (continued)

ADULT

	NATURE OF OPERATION	T	TS	C	A
8.	**Trigeminal and other Neuralgias**				
	Injection techniques/RF-lesion				
	Microvascular decompression				
	Others				
9.	**Stereotactic and Functional Neurosurgery**				
	Tumour biopsy				
	Seed implantation				
	Thalamotomy, Pallidotomy/Stimulation technique				
	Neuroablative procedures (chordotomy, DREZ)				
	Therapeutic electrostimulation (peripheral nerve, spinal)				
	Implantation of ports/pumps for intrathecal drug delivery				
	Others				
10.	**Surgery for Epilepsy**				
	Invasive diagnostic procedures (deep electrodes,grids,plates)				
	Temporal lobe resection				
	Extratemporal resection				
	Others				
11.	**Peripheral Nerve**				
	Entrapment decompression/transposition				
	Sutures (with graft)				
	Neurorhaphy				
	Sympathectomy				
	Brachial plexus repair				
	Tumour				
	Others				
12.	**Computer-aided Neurosurgical Planning (not the intervention)**				
13.	**Other Procedures (Please specify)**				

Table 2 (continued)

PAEDIATRIC (through 15 years)

	NATURE OF OPERATION	T	TS	C	A
1.	**Hydrocephalus and Congenital Malformation**				
	External ventricular drainage				
	Shunting procedure: initial				
	revision				
	Endoscopic fenestration				
	Arnold-Chiari/Dandy Walker				
	Encephalocele				
	Single sutural craniosynostosis				
	Complex craniosynostosis/ Craniofacial reconstruction				
2.	**Head and Spine Injuries**				
	Burr holes, ICP-monitoring/drainage/reservoir				
	Chronic subdural haematoma/hygroma				
	Extradural haematoma				
	Acute subdural haematoma				
	Acute intracerebral haematoma				
	Depressed fracture				
	Spinal trauma				
	Others				
3.	**Brain Tumours**				
	Supratentorial hemispheric tumours				
	Supratentorial midline tumours				
	Infratentorial tumours				
	Others				
4.	**Spine**				
	Meningo/meningomyelocele				
	Tethering syndromes				
	Tumour				
	Spinal dysraphism				
5.	**Functional**				
	Spasticity				
	Surgery for epilepsy				
6.	**Other Procedures (Please specify)**				

subspecialty areas of our specialty, particularly if one has to overlook the literature and work to scientific standards. However, a trainee during his training should see enough patients in all categories of the log-book to be able in recognition, in the diagnostic work-up, the differential diagnosis and the various forms of treatments of these diseases. He should be capable to inform the patient about the risks, the advantages, etc. of a certain treatment and he should be able and willing to refer the patient – if he does not perform the respective procedure with "adequate routine" – to a more experienced colleague or department.

One possible and recommended solution for the future is with all probability the development of subspecialty areas (as described in Chapter 16, G. Schackert) which may start during the last 1 or $1\frac{1}{2}$ years of the training programme.

During his training the resident should become familiar with all the techniques and procedures and should be able to handle those complex cases which he needs to know when choosing a subspecialty. A further deepening of the experiences and knowledge can then be acquired within the scope of an additional fellowship programme.

A second important question is how many procedures of each category must be performed during the training to reach "adequate routine" and competence.

The figures published in the UEMS neurosurgical part of the Training Charter are minimum figures and should be attained by every resident. Since residents have different abilities, ambition und capabilities, a competence range should be introduced. Thus a resident must at least receive the minimum competency in the respective area but may result in a much higher competence range. A very good description of the discussion on the operative total figures and the competence range is presented in one of the following chapters (K. W. Lindsay, Periodic Progress Evaluation).

Learning certainly does not stop at the end of a training programme but rather has to continue for the rest of life.

Correspondence: Prof. Dr. H.-J. Reulen, Schwojer Str. 19, 81249 München, Germany. e-mail: Ilona.Anders@med.uni-muenchen.de

Acta Neurochir (2004) [Suppl] 90: 67–71

Printed in Austria

IX Morbidity & mortality conferences – How can we do it?

J. Brennum[1] and **F. Gjerris**[2]

[1] The University Clinics of Neurosurgery, Copenhagen County Hospital, Glostrup, Denmark
[2] Rigshospitalet, Neuroscience Centre, Copenhagen, Denmark

Introduction

Quality assurance is a very important aspect of daily life in a neurosurgical department as well as an important parameter for the neurosurgical patient. Quality assurance programmes of some sort are common but still not implemented in all units. Some quality assurance programmes have been formulated as accreditation programmes to set a measure of good quality surgery [2], and have ended up in web site programmes [1]. In the near future such programmes [1] will play an increasing role, as the accreditation programmes sweep across Europe. However, quality assurance programmes, in which the performance of both the department in general and its individual members are analysed, are far more seldom. Imagine if airline pilots did not conduct debriefings of so-called near misses, situations that might have developed into a disaster. Or for that matter, if plane crashes did not automatically result in a full investigation. Would it make you feel safe, as a frequent flyer, if the pilot organisations and the airlines declared that these measures were no longer necessary due to the high ethical and moral standard of pilots in general, which in itself guarantees the best quality possible.

Some departments have implemented quality assurance or auditing systems [3, 4, 6, 7, 14, 16, 18] similar to those known in the airlines – *morbidity & mortality conferences*. Morbidity & mortality conferences seem to be more common in North America than in Europe. Morbidity & mortality conferences are well suited for any kind of department, be that University or general neurosurgical units [9, 12, 16, 18].

We have used morbidity & mortality conferences as an intricate part of our training programmes for a number of years, and found them to be an extremely helpful teaching tool.

Definition

By a morbidity & mortality conference we understand a conference within the individual department, or including a number of departments, as may for example be relevant for a trauma-receiving centre [7]. The conferences are based on real cases, i.e. near misses or plane crashes, from which it is possible for the individual staff member to learn and for the department to reflect upon its procedure relevant to the pertinent case. This means that the discussion covers "*what went wrong*" in the single case, "*what can we learn*" from the present case, where the problem may stem from part of the handling of the patient, i.e. history, diagnosis or operative activity. Now, having identified the source of the mishap, the next part of the learning process is to reflect upon "*what can we do better*" and "*how can we avoid the same mistake*" in the future?

Objective

Morbidity & mortality conferences may have many forms, but the common objective is to continuously improve the performance of the department, by improving the performance of its individual staff members and their collaboration. A way point towards this goal is to develop a foundation of trust and mutual confidence [6, 9, 10, 15, 17]. Hence, everybody should be encouraged to participate actively and open minded in these conferences. Even the slightest hint of a witch-hunt is extremely counterproductive and should be avoided [10].

Form

It is very important that the form of the morbidity & mortality conferences reflects the objective [11, 13, 14, 16]. The aim is not to denounce any members of the team or the staff but to allow everyone to take part in the discussion and learn from individual members mistakes or misjudgements. The trainees in neurosurgery, as in any other speciality, are for the vast majority young colleagues who are very eager to learn, and who aim to treat their patients as expertly as possible. There are lots of anxiety in being a young trainee and they need to know that their department will provide adequate supervision and training. They should not be harassed for not being as theoretically well founded as their trainers believe they themselves are. The trainees need a) to feel safe, b) to know that it is always acceptable to ask questions, c) that teaching is an elaborate part of the daily life in the department, and d) to know that in any patient's outcome, even a less favourable than expected, there may well be a lesson to learn.

Morbidity & mortality conferences may be viewed as a multipurpose tool that can be used as a quality assurance measurement, a teaching device and an opportunity for reflection, where protocols and procedures are reviewed, developed and improved. A good teaching neurosurgical department is not only a department full of theoretical and technically talented neurosurgeons but also a place with a scheduled and balanced training programme and regular teaching sessions and conferences. These are all valuable ingredients but in our way of thinking the most important foundation is the teaching culture and spirit within the department. The talented neurosurgical consultant may sometimes be the one in need of training, when it comes to the trade of teaching.

Structure

Morbidity & mortality conferences should be held on a regular basis. In our departments morbidity & mortality conferences are conducted once or twice a month. Morbidity & mortality conferences may have a variety of configurations:

- Review of all recent mortality cases since the last conference
- Review of all severe morbidity cases since the last conference
- Review of single cases
- Review of a couple of similar cases

We prefer one of the two latter forms because they allow us to choose different clinical subjects for the individual conferences. As stated previously, it is of utmost importance that the atmosphere of the morbidity & mortality conferences is that of a forum for mutual learning and not a place of finger pointing and punishment [7, 10]. This is not different from how the atmosphere and the teaching environment should be in the neurosurgical department in general.

One member of the staff, which may well be one of the trainees, presents a relevant summary of the pertinent case or cases, including demonstration of relevant images. Especially when morbidity & mortality conferences are introduced into the teaching programme of a department, it is prudent, at least in the beginning, to use anonymous cases [10]. This is simply done by using cases that are not recent, and by using transcripts from the patient charts, where any patient identifiers, dates and names or initials of doctors or nurses involved in the treatment are omitted. All this is done to get an objective, unbiased review of the case that is not contaminated with the urge to blame an individual or the urge to defend one's own action in the case.

The two first forms are also important, but they might be extremely time-consuming in very busy departments, for instance as in our departments with altogether up to 7,500 admissions and 4,500 operations per year.

It is our experience that the usage of anonymous cases makes everybody more open minded and receptive to learning. Once the morbidity and mortality conferences have become an accepted part of the teaching programme of the department and everybody recognises the merits of the conferences as mutual teaching experiences, there is no longer any need to maintain the use of anonymous cases. Furthermore, when the department has developed to a stage where it is generally accepted and expected that everybody comments on the performance of others with the aim to improve the general performance of the department, the resulting effect will be even greater. However, if you do not choose to use cases that are anonymous, it is important that the cases chosen for morbidity and mortality conferences are not selected only to reflect the practice of the more junior staff. The selection of cases should demonstrate that it is human and acceptable not to be perfect. What is not acceptable is not to learn from experience. If the selection of cases is biased towards demonstrating the mishaps of the junior staff, soon the feeling of being exposed and blamed is going to devaluate the teaching experience and replace it with fear [10].

In our department all head staff members participate in the identification of cases that are suitable for mortality & morbidity conferences. The director, the professor, or the head staff member responsible for the particular mortality & morbidity meeting, selects the cases to de demonstrated. Confidentiality is obviously very important. If the discussion of a case during a morbidity & mortality conference could have legal or other repercussions, the teaching value would be degraded, and it is likely that the morbidity & mortality conferences would altogether cease to exist.

To improve or elevate the learning experience, the staff member presenting the case should submit a short literature review or a specific scientific article relevant to the presented case or cases. The presentation itself should normally be brief, typically between 5 to 10 minutes, and the following 20 minutes should be used for open and free minded discussion of whether the diagnostic work up, treatment and care of the patient lived up to the expected standard of the department or whether the performance could have been better. If the consensus is that the performance of the department in the particular case did leave room for improvement, this then leads the discussion into the next phase. How can we improve the performance in future and avoid similar suboptimal performance? Should the case be reported to the Danish Patient Compensation Assurance System [8]? Sometimes the result of a morbidity & mortality conference is that a task force is formed to update the department's routine procedure book, based on the lessons learned. All doctors are informed of the final decisions. It is by no means necessary that the cases presented at a morbidity & mortality conference reflect mortality or severe morbidity, it may also be a brilliant way of demonstrating or exposing inefficient or obsolete procedures.

When morbidity & mortality conferences work at their best, they function both as a quality assurance process, a learning process, and as a cultural process in which the spirit of aiming towards mutual learning and improvement by openly sharing not only the success stories but also the problems and mistakes. Far more can be learned by analysing cases with morbidity and mortality than by analysing successful stories. The morbidity and mortality conferences are popular because they offer learning and opportunity to participate actively, independent of one's training level. Furthermore, they are popular because they are designed to be interactive and relevant, in contrast to the passive learning experience of a lecture.

Examples

In the following a couple of examples of recent morbidity & mortality conference cases are presented in abbreviated form, and the outcomes of those conferences are commented.

Example A

A 67-year-old man was admitted with a history typical of lumbar spinal canal stenosis, decreasing gait distance, and no paresis or sphincter disturbances. A stenosis at the L4/5 level was demonstrated by myelography, and he was treated with a laminectomy. Postoperatively, on the same day as the procedure, normal neurological function of the lower extremities was noted, but intermittent catheterisation was necessary. On the second day, the patient complained of a strange feeling in his feet, and intermittent catheterisation was still needed. The patient notes did not reveal whether any objective evaluation of patient was performed at this point in time. On the 8th day after surgery the patient was discharged with a catheter and a scheduled follow-up appointment at the department of urology. On the 12th post-surgical day the patient was readmitted because he still had a strange sensation in his legs and then had suffered several falls at home. A clinical investigation demonstrated that he had increased tone in his legs, bilateral extensive plantar responses, normal motor power, and slightly reduced touch sensation diffusely in his legs. An acute MRI demonstrated an extensive subdural haematoma reaching up to the mid-thoracic level.

Comments

Nobody at the morbidity & mortality conference had any trouble recognising the mistakes made in this case: On the second day a suspicion of a haematoma should have been raised, a clinical examination should have been performed and eventually relevant investigations made, i.e. an MRI. However, in our mind such a case serves as a far more powerful reminder of why all staff members have to be conscious in their evaluation of patients postoperatively than a scalding by the department chairman would have been.

Example B

A 72-year-old man was referred from the department of oncology with slight gait disturbances and back pain. He had a known history of colorectal cancer, operated 5 years previously. He had bilateral lung metastases and possible retroperitoneal metastases. A single level columnal pathological fracture at Th8 was demonstrated on MRI, with a wedge-shaped vertebra, with involvement of the most anterior part of the pedicles on both sides. The subarachnoidal space was obliterated at this leve, but the spinal cord was not deformed. The patient was found to have increased tone in his legs, normal sensation for touch, moderately reduced position sense and normal motor power and sphincter function. The patient was referred back to the department of oncology for acute radiotherapy. Over the following weeks the patient's lower extremity function deteriorated, and at this time a decompression and stabilization procedure was performed. This did not improve the function of the lower extremities and a few weeks later the patient was found to have multiple brain metastases.

Comments

This case led to a very interesting discussion of ethics and the role of the neurosurgeon in palliative treatment of the inevitably dying patient. Furthermore, this case led us to form a task force with the assignment to review and update our procedures for treatment of metastatic disease of spinal column, which was presented and discussed at a conference a month later.

Example C

A 37-year-old woman was admitted with a history typical of a one-sided acoustic schwannoma, confirmed by MRI. She was operated by a translabyrinthine approach without any operative complications. During the first day after operation she had no complaints at all but on the second day she slowly developed headache and vomiting, treated by medicine. The third day she demonstrated beginning unconsciousness, which was interpreted as caused by the given medicine. Early in the morning on the fourth day she became unconscious and an acute MRI disclosed a haematoma in the operative field and severe hydrocephalus. She was re-operated, but a fatal herniation had already occurred.

Comments

The case led to a many-sided discussion of the problems of post-operative observation by "too many different" doctors. Furthermore, the case led to an updated education of house officers in postoperative observation and repetitive courses in the most important symptoms and signs to be observed in patients following intracranial procedures.

Example D

A 42-year-old man was admitted with a typical history of long lasting lumbar pain and a shorter one of one-sided radicular symptoms and signs of a lumbar disc herniation, confirmed by MRI at the level of the 4th lumbar disc. He was operated with a classical one-sided lumbar approach. After the operation the symptoms were only slightly improved but in spite of this he was dismissed. At the postoperative control in the outpatient clinic three months later, the patient said that the preoperative symptoms had returned within two weeks of the operation, and had been unchanged since. A control X-ray disclosed, that the patient had been operated at a wrong level. The patient was re-operated, but some of the symptoms remained.

Comments

During the mortality and morbidity conference the general rules for spinal operations were discussed. The internal investigations showed that the surgeon did not follow the instructions of the clinics, which clearly stated that a peri-operative X-ray confirmation of the height is the gold standard. A discussion followed concerning the problem of casual post-operative observation by "too many different doctors" versus the problem of potentially biased postoperative observations, when these only are performed by the surgeon. It was decided to make a notification to the Danish patient compensation insurance company [8]. Finally, it was debated how procedures at a wrong level could be avoided and later again this was discussed in a more scientific forum [5].

Conclusion

We regularly use such cases to adjust behaviour. The insight gained by the individual member of the staff of their role or potential role in the outcome of cases like the ones above is an eye-opener. Of course the first one was not the result of everybody "not bothering" but reflected an extremely busy week in the department during a holiday, where corners were cut to make ends meet. If cases like these are addressed by lecturing the staff about "their irresponsible and poor performance", this will put everybody in a defensive mode, justifying their actions with the workload etc. When cases like number one and three were presented at the morbidity & mortality conference, the result was that everybody felt sorry for the patients and acknowledged the need to improve and maintain a high standard of postoperative evaluation of patients. To maintain a high standard of postoperative evaluation, another morbidity & mortality conference may be used as a booster, if the quality of postoperative evaluations declines again.

We have found the morbidity & mortality conference to be of great value in our departments, both as a teaching tool and as a tool to modify clinical behaviour and the culture of the department. The morbidity & mortality conferences have made it more acceptable to comment on and discuss each other's performance for the benefit of the patients without antagonising each other. In our opinion morbidity and mortality conferences should be part of the daily life in a neurosurgical department.

References

1. Agency for Healthcare Research and Quality. AHRQ WebM&M. *www.webmm.ahrq.gov*
2. Ashbaugh DG, Lung JA (1977) Benefits of an intensive community surgical audit program. Arch Surg 112: 389–390
3. Berthold LD, Hoppe M, Konig H, Saar B, Wagner HJ, Lorenz W, Klose KJ (1998) Mortalitats- und Morbiditatskonferenz in der Radiologie. [Mortality and morbidity conference in radiology]. Rofo Fortschr Geb Rontgenstr Neuen Bildgeb Verfahr 169: 585–589
4. Biddle C (1991) The morbidity and mortality conference: a prolegomenon on its role as an anesthesia risk-management tool. Nurse Anesth 2: 165–171
5. Degn J, Gjerris F (2004) Operation against lumbar disc prolapse. Is it possible to avoid a wrong level? (Operation for lumbal diskusprolaps. Kan indgreb på forkert niveau forebygges? (In Danish)) Ugeskr Læger 166: 1757–1759
6. Eckel HE, Streppel M, Schmalenbach K, Volling P, Schrappe M, Dietz A, Bootz F (2000) Qualitätsicherung in der HNO-Tumorchirurgie. HNO 48: 902–910
7. Esselman PC, Dillman Long J (2002) Morbidity and management conference: an approach to quality improvement in brain injury rehabilitation. J Head Trauma Rehab 17: 257–262
8. Gjerris F, Grünfeld A (1996) Patients insurance and compensation policy in Denmark and other Scandinavian countries. Invited Lecture at the "European Conference on Neurosurgery and Public Health". WHO, Madrid, Spain
9. Harbison SP, Regehr G (1999) Faculty and resident opinions regarding the role of morbidity and mortality conference. Am J Surg 177: 136–139
10. Hobgood CD, Ma OJ, Swart GL (2000) Emergency medicine resident errors: identification and educational utilization. Acad Emerg Med 7: 1317–1320
11. Hoyt DB (1997) Clinical practice guidelines. Am J Surg 173: 32–34
12. Ku Y, Tominaga M, Iwasaki T, Fukumoto T, Suzuki Y, Fujino Y, Hori Y, Kuroda Y (2000) Chairpersons' opinions regarding quality control of surgical faculty performance in Japanese academic surgery departments. Am J Surg 180: 46–50
13. Murayama KM, Derossis AM, DaRosa DA, Sherman HB, Fryer JP (2002) A critical evaluation of the morbidity and mortality conference. Am J Surg 183: 246–250
14. O'Connell PR, Kirwan WO, Brady MP, O'Donnell JA (1988) Surgical audit: the value of a morbidity and mortality conference. Ir J Med Sci 157: 100–103
15. Orlander JD, Barber TW, Fincke BG (2002) The morbidity and mortality conference: the delicate nature of learning from error. Acad Med 77: 1001–1006
16. Seiler RW (2001) Principles of the morbidity and mortality conference. Acta Neurochir (Wien) [Suppl] 78: 125–126
17. Thompson JS, Prior MA (1992) Quality assurance and morbidity and mortality conference. J Surg Res 52: 97–100
18. Zubarik R, Eisen G, Mastropietro C, Lopez J, Carroll J, Benjamin S, Fleischer DE (1999) Prospective analysis of complications 30 days after outpatient upper endoscopy. Am J Gastroenterol 94: 1539–1545

Correspondence: J. Brennum, The University Clinic of Neurosurgery, Copenhagen County Hospital, DK-2600, Glostrup, Denmark. e-mail: brennum@dadlnet.dk

Acta Neurochir (2004) [Suppl] 90: 73–76

Printed in Austria

X Problem-based learning in residency training and the tutorial process for training and education in neurosurgery

P. A. Winkler and **J.-C. Tonn**

Department of Neurosurgery, Klinikum Großhadern, Ludwig-Maximilians-University of Munich, Munich, Germany

Introduction

The educational climate in more traditional, didactic educational settings in neurosurgery, at least in Europe, works against "facilitatory tutorial teaching" of the residents in neurosurgery. In these settings, the resident and fellow is typically expected to know the right answer. S/he learned a long time ago that it is best to stay silent if s/he does not know the answer, or is unsure of it, for s/he fears that s/he may blame himself when being wrong with an answer. An admission of not knowing something would be used as evidence of inadequate study or lack of knowledge. Unless a resident has been in a more liberal or alternative high school or university, this climate has usually been in existence throughout his educational career, from kindergarten on [3].

The actual personnel and financial requirements necessitate a careful and economical application of the available resources, in this particular situation the teaching resources. "Facilitatory tutorial teaching" describes a culture of teaching in which a constructive atmosphere under the supervision of an experienced tutor is created.

At the anglo-saxon universities the title "tutor" is usually associated with someone who takes up the position of a teacher or master. Although the term "tutor" may therefore not be ideal for a teacher employing a facilitatory or Socratic teaching, respectively, style, it has become commonly used in this way. As "tutorial process" the interaction between the tutor and a "small group" of trainees with a maximum of eight group members is defined [1, 2]. The ability and, with increasing experience the skills of the tutor to use facilitatory teaching during the group learning process is the major determinant of the quality and the success of any educational method. Tutoring is a teaching skill central to problem-based, self-directed learning. Several universities and national societies offer "tutoring" and "facilitatory teaching" in form of a course for trainers to prepare them in modern teaching. It would be wise, if the EANS in future would also develop courses for training in modern teaching techniques.

How can we apply such teaching techniques in the clinical environment? In the daily practice of neurosurgery it is logical to combine the admission examination and the discussion about the best management of the patient with a problem-based, case-oriented learning for the residents and fellows. Basically, this technique can be applied during all forms of teaching, in conferences, seminars etc.

The intent of this book chapter is to present a conceptual basis for facilitatory teaching, making this new method of learning easier to understand, as well as to present practical suggestions how to develop and practise these skills with time. Over the last ten years, the first author of this book chapter had the opportunity to practise this style of teaching in seminars of neuroanatomy for second-year-students (here combined with conventional didactic methods), in courses of clinical neurosurgery for fifth-year-students and in a residency-training program.

The case presentation

As a vehicle of learning, the daily case should be used to initiate and drive the teaching process. Depending on the level of knowledge a straight forward case or a more complex case can be selected. This decision preferably is made by the tutor. Decision points elicit intellectual commitment, and help to raise the level of inquiry [4]. Given the busy daily time schedule a specific time period should be preserved each day for case presentation and discussion. It seems that the possibly best time is after the "core activities" in the operating theatre and the work on the ward. "The case" is best presented by a member of the small group, a trainee or a student, who during the day had the opportunity to interview and examine the patient meticulously under supervision. Beginning with the vital characteristics of the patient, (i.e. vital status, chief complaint, history of the present illness, pertinent past medical history, social and family history, physical exam, labs and diagnostic studies, treatments, etc.), actual problems of the patient and neuroradiological imaging-presentation, a whole picture of the suspected disease has to be described. For this procedure 8 out of 40 minutes of the whole teaching session are reserved.

Only if the tutor and the group have received all relevant data, the process can continue. If not, the tutor has to take care that this information is supplied. Next, the trainee continues with the discussion of the differential diagnosis, the disease etiology, its natural history, appropriate therapeutic options, neurosurgical procedures and approaches, its outcome and complications. At this point, the skilled tutor animates the other group members to take part in the discussion:

- Does everybody agree with the statements made?
- Are the conclusions adequate?
- Are there alternative therapeutic options, etc.?

The tasks of the tutor

The tutor has to find the right balance as a facilitator of the learning process. He asks questions, activates the group members to become involved, but he should not provide the desired information himself. The tutor's function aims at developing the residents' thinking or reasoning skills (problem solving, metacognition, critical thinking) and at helping to become independent, self-directed learners.

The term "*metacognition*" describes aspects like thought, reflection and deliberation. Metacognition is the executive function in thinking: pondering, deliberating, or reflecting on a problem or situation; reviewing what is known about the problem at hand; creating hypotheses; making decisions about what observations to make and what questions to ask; questioning the meaning of new information obtained from inquiry; evaluating other sources of information; reflecting on and reviewing what has been learned, what it all may mean and what needs to be done next.

Anyone who does not use metacognitive skills when faced with new and difficult problems is an impulsive thinker, someone who operates on reflex behaviours, guesses or hunches (i.e. without thinking). This is the trainee we all dread and the professional from whom we would prefer not to receive a service.

The tutor must carefully guide the respective trainee but also the whole group through all the steps of the particular learning process. The tutor should carefully guide trainee and group through analysis and synthesis. If action steps or solutions for a problem are to be undertaken, the group must entertain alternatives and consider the pros and cons, for instance the pros and cons for a stabilisation/instrumentation in a specific case. The tutor should be certain that all the appropriate steps are thoroughly covered. Particularly if a complex problem is to be analysed, the tutor must be sure the trainee structures the problem and goes through all stages of the hypothetico-deductive process.

A further task of the tutor is to keep the discussion process moving, to make sure that no essential part of the case evaluation is passed over or neglected and that the phases are addressed in the right sequence. For example, the tutor should be certain that all possible hypotheses or explanations for the cause of the problem are explored before he allows the group to go on with the next step.

The tutor should never let ideas, terms, explanations or comments go unchallenged or undefined. Anytime a scientific term, label or eponym is used, the trainee should be asked to define the term. The tutor cannot assume that a trainee correctly understands a concept or entity because he can use the label correctly. With the discussion going on the tutor gains a pretty good impression of the trainee's knowledge and understanding of the particular case. If necessary, he may ask some questions until the trainee has come to the depth of knowledge expected of him or her.

An important task is to involve all trainees in the group work. If the final solutions and decisions are made more or less as a consensus in the group, this is not only a reward but also an important experience for the participants. To facilitate the interchange between trainees, the tutor has to avoid to become the focal point of the discussions. If s/he is not careful, s/he will find that each trainee is answering only his/her questions and that each trainee is addressing the tutor in the discussions and not each other. Instead of a working group, the tutor will have five or six individuals, each interacting only with the tutor.

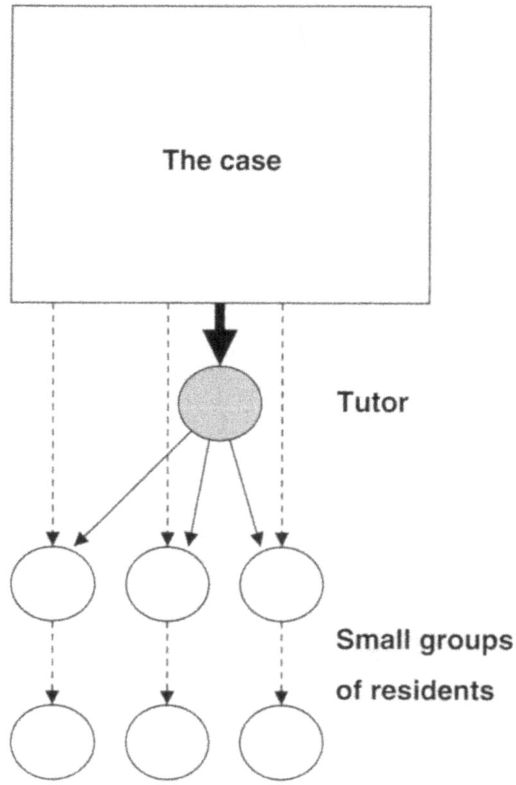

Fig. 1. Conventional teaching style

Interpersonal dynamics as a challenge for the tutor

Occasionally "*interpersonal dynamics*" may arise in the group. Silence, late arrival, sarcasm, lack of individual productivity, lack of initiative, personal instead of objective arguments, trainees taking sides on an issue, expressions of dissatisfaction with learning or attempts by a trainee to take over in the group should be recognized as important symptoms. When such problems become apparent to the tutor, it is best to approach them at a metacognitive level, i.e. at the level of objective, unprejudiced and unbiased decision makings. The two basic challenges for a tutor in small group learning are attending the group's educational progress at the metacognitive level and the group's interpersonal dynamics. If the tutor appreciates that s/he is the trainee's metacognitive conscience, his or her specific teaching role becomes more understandable.

Architecture of the small group learning process

It is important to form small groups consisting of the responsible tutor (consultants, subspecialists) and the trainees (residents, fellows, students, guests). The number of participants, however, should not exceed eight (8!) persons (Figs. 1 and 2).

In the clinical setting, either the assigned trainer works with his team on a regular schedule or a subspecialist works with all residents once a week and teaches a particular pathology. Even a combination of both is possible. If this is done on a regular basis, the trainees certainly will acquire a high competence in problem solving.

Summary of the general principles for tutorial teaching

Every responsible consultant or staff member who functions as a tutor should follow the subsequent "ten laws":

1. It is essential that the tutor avoids expressing a deprecatory opinion concerning the correctness or quality of any trainee's comments or contributions.
2. The tutor should push the trainee to a deeper level of understanding.
3. Discussions between trainees, comments and critical analysis of each other's ideas or knowledge must always be encouraged.
4. All decisions should be by group consensus. The tutor must be certain that all trainees contribute to the final decision.
5. The tutor should do whatever is necessary to get the trainees to talk and discuss among themselves.
6. Questions, particularly like "Are you sure you're right?" or "Are you comfortable with that decision?" should be asked to trainees when they are correct as often as when, in the mind of the tutor, they are incorrect in their opinions and statements.
7. The tutor should determine the goal of the specific session.
8. The tutor must monitor whether this goal has been reached and whether a trainee has made an educational progress.

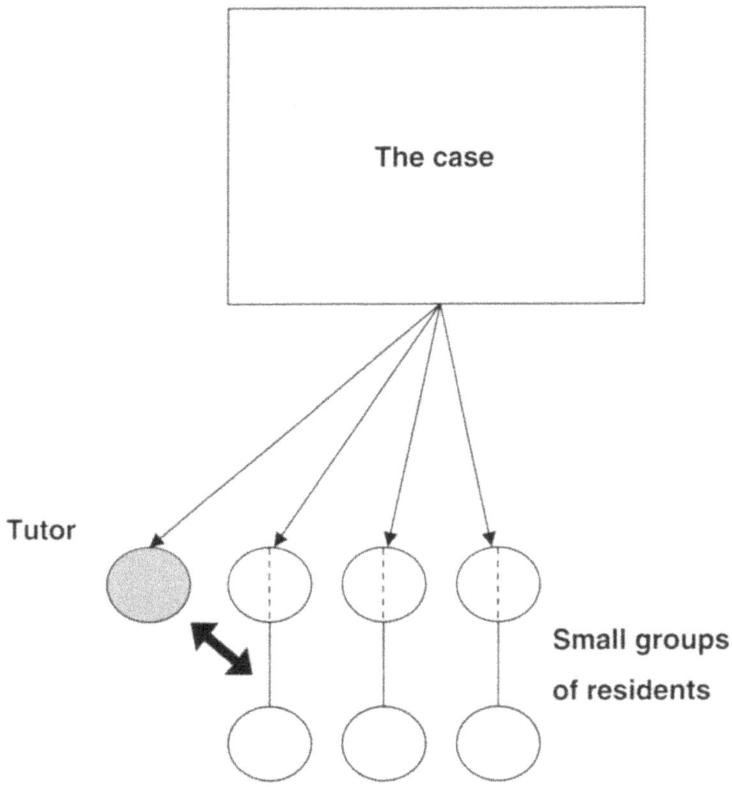

Fig. 2. Problem based learning and the tutorial process

9. The tutor needs to be aware of potential interpersonal problems in the group and make the interventions necessary to maintain an effective group process.
10. None of these tutorial activities should become the sole task of the tutor. The tutor must constantly work toward getting the group of trainees to take on the responsibility for the group learning process.

Conclusions

The tutor is responsible for the process of neurosurgical trainees' learning. S/he facilitates the trainees' learning through guidance at the metacognitive level. The small group-tutorial process should provide trainees with the metacognitive skills they will need to do this – as they acquire the skills to learn in contexts and practices relevant to their future.

Acknowledgement

The authors deeply acknowledge and thank Prof. Tom Aretz from Harvard-Medical-School in Boston for his valuable help in correcting and revising the manuscript.

References

1. Albanese MA, Mitchell S (1993) Problem based learning: (a review of literature on its outcomes and implementation issues. Acad Med 68: 1–48
2. Armstrong EG (1997) A hybrid model of problem based learning. In: Boud D, Feletti G (eds) The challenge of problem based learning, 2nd edn. London, Kogan Page 14: 137–150
3. Barrows HS (1992) The tutorial process, revised edn. Southern Illinois University School of Medicine, Springfield, Illinois
4. Glick TH, Armstrong EG (1996) Crafting cases for problem-based learning: experience in a neuroscience course. Med Educ 30: 24–30

Correspondence: Peter A. Winkler, Department of Neurosurgery, Klinikum Großhadern, Ludwig-Maximilians-University of Munich, Marchioninistr. 15, Munich, Germany. e-mail: pwinkler@nc.med.uni-muenchen.de

Acta Neurochir (2004) [Suppl] 90: 77–95

Printed in Austria

XI Periodic progress evaluation

K. W. Lindsay

Department of Neurosurgery, Southern General Hospital, Glasgow, UK

Introduction

Successful completion of neurosurgical training requires that trainees attain a variety of skills (Table 1) of which technical competence and judgement are perhaps the most critically important. But how do we evaluate these skills? How do we ensure that trainees satisfactorily progress throughout their training? How do we ensure that after a specified number of years trainees have achieved sufficient competence to permit safe neurosurgical practice? Too often such decisions depend on the subjective impressions of the clinical teachers. These may be reliable, particularly if based upon the consensus view of a large number of observers – but does this always apply? Does adequate documentation of the trainees' progress or failure always exist? It is no longer acceptable for trainees to complete training and be deemed 'competent' without undergoing some form of formal assessment. Yet to obtain a valid, objective and reliable method of assessing competence in these numerous skills, which remains feasible in terms of human and physical resources, presents a formidable challenge.

Table 1. *Competencies required in neurosurgical training*

Medical skills	
Knowledge of basic neurosciences	
Knowledge of clinical skills	– examination
	interpretation of symptoms/signs
	making a diagnosis
	treatment options
Decision making	
Surgical skills/manual dexterity	
Application of knowledge to clinical practice	
Communication skills	
Establish patient/clinician relationship	
History taking	
Relay information to the health care team	
Obtain consent	
Communicate bad news/bereavement	
Teaching/learning skills	
Critically appraise medical information incl. research	
Develop continual self education	
Pass on knowledge and skills to others	
Personal effectiveness	
Consult effectively with other clinicians	
Contribute to teamwork	
Use time effectively	
Management	
Utilise and prioritise available resources within healthcare organisation	
Utilise information technology	

In 1997, a task force charged with reporting on "Clinical Academic Careers" recommended that the Royal Colleges "give serious consideration to establishing innovated procedures, other than the written examination, to assess clinical competence of candidates for the Certificate of Completion of Specialist Training (CCST), rather than just time spent" [8]. In response to this the Surgical Royal Colleges set up working parties and committees to look into the issues involved, but progress has been slow.

In this chapter I will describe the methods used in the UK in the last decade to assess progress through neurosurgical training and will discuss their limitations. I will also review other methods, presently under consideration, which attempt to determine more objectively whether or not the trainee has achieved a satisfactory level of competence.

Progress evaluation – process and timing

Evaluation of progress of a trainee takes place at two levels, firstly at a local level by the trainers, by the Training Programme Director and by the Postgraduate Dean (the statutory source of trainee funding) and secondly, at a National level (for the UK and Ireland) by the Specialist Advisory Committee (SAC) in Neurosurgery acting on behalf of the Joint Committee for Higher Surgical Training (JCHST) of the Surgical Royal Colleges.

Local evaluation

Assessments occur at *6 months, one year and annually* thereafter. The *trainee assessment form* (Appendix I and II) forms the basis of these progress assessments. All trainers supervising training complete a form at the above periods or on completion of a training placement, if this is of less than one year's duration, taking into account the years of training already completed. The forms attempt to cover the range of required skills and include the trainees' capability of recording and conveying patient details of history, examination and investigative findings to senior staff, consenting patients for operative procedures, communicating with patients and relatives and passing on distressing information (e.g., malignancy or death) in a sensitive, caring manner. For each criterion, they categorise the trainee as – satisfactory, *or* needing targeted training in an area *or* unsatisfactory, needing to repeat training in this area.

The trainer produces a written summary and indicates whether

- training is satisfactory in all aspects permitting the trainee to proceed to the next stage of the programme,
- any areas of weakness have been identified requiring correction at the next placement,
- training must be repeated *or*
- the trainee should be counselled by the Postgraduate Dean/Programme Director about choosing an alternative career pathway.

The trainers discuss their conclusions with the trainee, who is asked to add comments and to sign the form (to confirm that he has seen, but not necessarily agreed with the conclusions).

A very similar form, modified by H. J. Reulen is available from the Joint Residency Advisory and Accreditation Committee of the EANS/UEMS (see web site EANS).

The *assessment panel*, composed of at least four members including the Training Programme Director, the Postgraduate Dean's representative and at least one other trainer, meets annually and interviews all trainees on the training programme to ascertain achievements and progress. The panel reviews the

- Training portfolio which includes an up to date *curriculum vitae* incorporating –
  - (i) details of previous training posts, dates, duration and trainers.
  - (ii) details of examinations passed e.g. MRCS
  - (iii) list of publications with copies of published first page/abstract.
  - (iv) list of research presentations at local, national and international meetings.
  - (v) list of courses attended.
  - (vi) updated cumulative operative totals (see Chapter VI)
  - (vii) copies of assessment forms for the end of each training year, completed and signed by both trainers and trainee.
- Trainee assessment form
- Neurosurgical logbook

and makes a final decision regarding progression to the next training placement.

Prior to the interview, the trainee also completes and submits a *training post assessment form* (Appendix III) commenting on any perceived deficiencies in the training programme related to clinical training, the workload, teaching and supervision in theatre, research support, feedback of progress and career advice. The panel can discuss any items of concern with the trainee. Where possible, the Training Programme Director would be responsible for correcting any such deficiencies. Completed assessment forms are sent to the central Specialist Advisory Committee in Neurosurgery. Forms indicating a significant problem in training may trigger an interview with this committee (see below).

Right of appeal

If the trainee disagrees with any decision, he or she has the right of appeal to the assessment panel. If asked to repeat training or to withdraw from the programme, the trainee has the right of appeal to an appeals panel, chaired by the Postgraduate Dean, that excludes any member of the original assessment panel.

National level evaluation

Two members of the Specialist Advisory Committee (SAC) interview trainees in their third year of training, or more frequently if any significant problems arise. Before each interview, trainees complete a short structured information sheet providing details on weekly timetable, operative experience and supervision, the on-call rota, the academic programme, research, and administrative duties. They also present their cumulative operative totals for review. The interviewers report their findings back to the whole committee. If the SAC believes any deficiencies exist the Training Programme Director is notified.

Two SAC members visit every training programme once every four years to monitor standards and quality of training. As well as inspecting facilities and reviewing the trainees' workload, the visitors interview all trainees on the programme, irrespective of their year of training.

End of training assessment

At the end of a *minimum of 6 years* of training the trainee applies to the SAC for recommendation for the Certificate of Completion of Specialist Training (CCST). To succeed, the trainee should have

- completed 5 years of clinical neurosurgical training and one in research or any other branch of the specialty,
- obtained satisfactory assessments at the end of each year,
- maintained a logbook (Chapter VI), validated by his trainers, showing that he or she has assisted in a wide variety of cases, including those performed personally, those assisted by a trainer or more senior trainee, and those where the trainee acted as assistant,
- a cumulative list of operative totals for each procedure, indicating that these approach the median figure for the majority of procedures (see chapter VII, Table 1),
- passed the Intercollegiate Board Examination in Neurosurgery,
- received a reference from all trainers indicating a satisfactory performance.

The SAC scrutinises the above information and tries to ensure that no deficiencies exist. In a proportion, recommendation for the CCST award is deferred.

Progress evaluation – methods

In-training evaluation

Trainers (i.e. consultants or specialists) working directly with the trainee for months or years should be capable of providing a meaningful judgement of his or her abilities. But such observations, although perhaps accurate, are inevitably based on subjective assessment rather than objective facts. The *trainee assessment form* provides a structured format, compelling trainers to consider trainees' abilities for individual skills, but the available categories may fail to discriminate between trainees of varying ability. Completion of assessment forms by multiple trainers for any one trainee must help to improve validity but other methods should be sought.

Operative totals

The trainee logbooks and summative operative totals go some way toward providing a more objective method of assessment. These detail operative experience, and this in turn should indirectly reflect operative skills. Trainers will more readily permit trainees to perform procedures if they are confident of the trainees' abilities. The number of procedures performed for any one condition will reflect the likelihood that the trainee will have experienced complications and difficulties that might arise for that condition. Operative totals are simple to monitor by the trainer and by the local and national training committees. The national training committee (the SAC) can set minimal targets for certain key procedures and encourage trainees to achieve median values for the majority of procedures.

Using operative totals to monitor competence requires some caution –

- The numbers of procedures performed personally by the trainees and the numbers when the consultant has actively assisted may depend to some extent on the personality of the trainer and the extent of supervision he or she imposes.
- A degree of variability may exist in the way the trainee categorizes his or her participation in the

procedure. This depends to some extent on the integrity of the trainee, unless the trainer checks and countersigns every procedure (for categories and redefinitions see Chapter VII).

- Performing many operative procedures does not necessarily mean that the trainee has received good training; nor does it ensure that the procedures were performed well. Operative training should progress through various stages – the trainee assisting the trainer, the trainer assisting, the trainer observing scrubbed, the trainer observing unscrubbed, and finally with the trainer available but not in the operating theatre. Some countries (e.g., Germany) require that the trainer be present in the operating theatre for the whole procedure, but this deprives the experienced trainee of the opportunity to gain the self-confidence required for independent practice. Scrutiny of the logbook for numbers of procedures "assisted by the trainer" ensures that the appropriate training steps have been followed.
- If a training committee set a target number of procedures, the danger would be that trainees spend their time chasing operative numbers rather than ensuring that they obtain a balanced neurosurgical training. This criticism may apply, but most would accept that, along with judgment, operative ability is the most crucial aspect of neurosurgical training.

Operative competencies

Recording operative totals provides a limited measure of competence. To seek alternative methods of evaluating progress, the SAC in Neurosurgery proposed taking operative competencies a step further. Trainees in conjunction with their trainers would categorize their operative abilities for each procedure into one of four grades, as follows: *(A) not able to perform the procedure; (B) competent to perform the procedure with direct supervision; (C) competent to perform the procedure without direct supervision; and (D) competent to deal with complications and difficulties that may arise.* These competencies would be recorded at three stages in training: at the end of the second year, at the end of the fourth year, and at the end of the sixth year [4]. The SAC has drawn up three tables indicating the minimal competency expected at these three stages (Table 2 a,b,c). At each stage, the trainee would tabulate his/her cumulative operative totals and perceived level of competence and the trainers and the Training Programme Director would validate the completed forms.

Although training in the UK aims to produce a neurosurgeon 'capable of independent practice', it is not expected that trainees attain competence in every operative procedure (although trainees should have sufficient expertise to care for the patient until referral to an appropriate neurosurgeon is arranged). Table 2c illustrates those procedures where the SAC would expect operative competence to be developed *after* completion of training (even though the trainee undertook a subspecialisation year in the field). Such procedures would include

- complex basal meningiomas,
- transphenoidal micro-adenomas,
- acoustic neuromas
- complex arteriovenous malformations,
- paediatric neurosurgical procedures other than shunt insertion/revision.
- intradural intramedullary spinal tumours
- functional neurosurgery

Another method of assessing technical skills under consideration, is that described for general surgical procedures by Winckel et al. [9]. This involves defining a few core procedures and creating a Structured Technical Skills Assessment Form (STSAF) which consists of two parts. In the first part a checklist divides the procedure into numerous components e.g. positioning on the table, incision, use of cautery, exposure, use of the microscope, dural opening, achievement of the procedure, closure, postoperative care etc. A trained evaluator assesses the trainee's capability of performing each step. The second part of the form assesses global skills e.g. respect for tissues, instrument handling, flow of procedure, understanding of surgical anatomy, use of assistants etc. Winckel et al. found high inter-rater reliability with this technique. The checklists also competently distinguished between junior and senior trainees.

Reznick's team also developed an objective method to test surgical skills using 'bench models' to simulate different stages within a surgical procedures (e.g. bowel anastomosis) [5, 7]. Again the authors created a structured form – the Objective Structured Assessment of Surgical Skills (OSATS) has been created with checklists evaluating ability at performing individual steps and a 'global rating scale' including the skills listed above, looking at surgical 'behaviour'. These

Table 2 (a). *Expected competencies – end of 2nd year*

NEUROSURGICAL TRAINING Name: Date:

OPERATIVE COMPETENCIES - END OF 2nd YEAR
A = Not able to perform procedure
B = Competent to perform procedure under direct supervision
C = Competent to perform procedure without direct supervision
D = Competent to deal with complications and difficulties which may arise

Cumulative operative totals
P = No direct supervision
SU = Trainer in theatre
SS = Trainer scrubbed
A = Assisting trainer

		A	B	C	D	P	SU	SS	A
Basic techniques	Burrhole insertion								
	Craniotomy								
Head Injuries:	craniotomy - extradural								
	craniotomy - acute subdural								
	craniotomy - intracerebral								
	depressed fractures								
	burr hole - chronic subdural								
Supratentorial tumours:	stereotactic/ids biopsy								
	craniotomy - intrinsic tumour								
	meningioma - vault								
	meningioma - parasagittal								
	meningioma - complex basal								
Midline tumours	transphenoidal macroadenoma								
	transphenoidal microadenoma								
Post. fossa tumours	malignant								
	acoustic								
Hydrocephalus	external ventricular drain								
	shunts insertion								
	shunt revision								
Neuroendoscopy									
Vascular	craniotomy - aneurysm								
	craniotomy - AVM								
	craniotomy - intracerebral haematoma								
	posterior fossa haematoma								
Spine	cervical disc disease / spondylosis								
	thoracic disc disease								
	lumbar disc disease/spondylosis								
	tumours - extradural								
	tumours - intradural extramedullary								
	tumours - intradural intramedullary								
	spinal fixation								
Pain:	trigeminal neuralgia - lesion								
	trigeminal neuralgia - MVD								
PAEDIATRIC									
Head injuries	haematoma								
	chronic subdural/hygroma								
	depressed fracture								
	ICP monitoring								
Tumours	supratentorial								
	infratentorial								
	stereotactic / ids biopsy								
Hydrocephalus	external ventricular drain								
	shunt insertion/revision								
	Arnold Chiari								
	Neuroendoscopy								
Spine	mening/meningomyelocele								
	tethering syndromes								
Paediatric functional	spasticity								
	surgery for epilepsy								
Craniofacial	sutural craniectomy								
	combined craniofacial								
	encephalocele								

[shaded box] - minimal competency

Table 2 (b). *Expected competencies – end of 4th year*

NEUROSURGICAL TRAINING	Name:				Date:				
OPERATIVE COMPETENCIES - END OF 4th YEAR A = Not able to perform procedure B = Competent to perform procedure under direct supervision C = Competent to perform procedure without direct supervision D = Competent to deal with complications and difficulties which may arise						Cumulative operative totals P = No direct supervision SU = Trainer in theatre SS = Trainer scrubbed A = Assisting trainer			
		A	B	C	D	P	SU	SS	A
Basic techniques	Burrhole insertion								
	Craniotomy								
Head Injuries:	craniotomy - extradural								
	craniotomy - acute subdural								
	craniotomy - intracerebral								
	depressed fractures								
	burr hole - chronic subdural								
Supratentorial tumours:	stereotactic/ids biopsy								
	craniotomy - intrinsic tumour								
	meningioma - vault								
	meningioma - parasagittal								
	meningioma - complex basal								
Midline tumours	transphenoidal macroadenoma								
	transphenoidal microadenoma								
Post. fossa tumours	malignant								
	acoustic								
Hydrocephalus	external ventricular drain								
	shunts insertion								
	shunt revision								
Neuroendoscopy									
Vascular	craniotomy - aneurysm								
	craniotomy - AVM								
	craniotomy - intracerebral haematoma								
	posterior fossa haematoma								
Spine	cervical disc disease / spondylosis								
	thoracic disc disease								
	lumbar disc disease/spondylosis								
	tumours - extradural								
	tumours - intradural extramedullary								
	tumours - intradural intramedullary								
	spinal fixation								
Pain:	trigeminal neuralgia - lesion								
	trigeminal neuralgia - MVD								
PAEDIATRIC									
Head injuries	haematoma								
	chronic subdural/hygroma								
	depressed fracture								
	ICP monitoring								
Tumours	supratentorial								
	infratentorial								
	stereotactic / ids biopsy								
Hydrocephalus	external ventricular drain								
	shunt insertion/revision								
	Arnold Chiari								
	Neuroendoscopy								
Spine	mening/meningomyelocele								
	tethering syndromes								
Paediatric functional	spasticity								
	surgery for epilepsy								
Craniofacial	sutural craniectomy								
	combined craniofacial								
	encephalocele								

[shaded box] - minimal competency

Table 2 (c). *Expected competencies – end of 6th year*

NEUROSURGICAL TRAINING Name: Date:

OPERATIVE COMPETENCIES - END OF 6th YEAR
A = Not able to perform procedure
B = Competent to perform procedure under direct supervision
C = Competent to perform procedure without direct supervision
D = Competent to deal with complications and difficulties which may arise

Cumulative operative totals
P = No direct supervision
SU = Trainer in theatre
SS = Trainer scrubbed
A = Assisting trainer

		A	B	C	D	P	SU	SS	A
Basic techniques	Burrhole insertion								
	Craniotomy								
Head Injuries:	craniotomy - extradural								
	craniotomy - acute subdural								
	craniotomy - intracerebral								
	depressed fractures								
	burr hole - chronic subdural								
Supratentorial tumours:	stereotactic/ids biopsy								
	craniotomy - intrinsic tumour								
	meningioma - vault								
	meningioma - parasagittal								
	meningioma - complex basal								
Midline tumours	transphenoidal macroadenoma								
	transphenoidal microadenoma								
Post. fossa tumours	malignant								
	acoustic								
Hydrocephalus	external ventricular drain								
	shunts insertion								
	shunt revision								
Neuroendoscopy									
Vascular	craniotomy - aneurysm								
	craniotomy - AVM								
	craniotomy - intracerebral haematoma								
	posterior fossa haematoma								
Spine	cervical disc disease / spondylosis								
	thoracic disc disease								
	lumbar disc disease/spondylosis								
	tumours - extradural								
	tumours - intradural extramedullary								
	tumours - intradural intramedullary								
	spinal fixation								
Pain:	trigeminal neuralgia - lesion								
	trigeminal neuralgia - MVD								
PAEDIATRIC									
Head injuries	haematoma								
	chronic subdural/hygroma								
	depressed fracture								
	ICP monitoring								
Tumours	supratentorial								
	infratentorial								
	stereotactic / ids biopsy								
Hydrocephalus	external ventricular drain								
	shunt insertion/revision								
	Arnold Chiari								
	Neuroendoscopy								
Spine	mening/meningomyelocele								
	tethering syndromes								
Paediatric functional	spasticity								
	surgery for epilepsy								
Craniofacial	sutural craniectomy								
	combined craniofacial								
	encephalocele								

[shaded box] - minimal competency

appear to correlate with the trainers' opinions about trainees' progress in the operating theatre. However to create such facilities on a wide scale basis would be labour-intensive and expensive and Reznick's techniques do not apply to neurosurgical practice. Similar assessment devices provide objective measurements of economy of motion and number of movements of laparoscopic surgical instruments using both real and virtual reality [2], but again such techniques are not applicable to neurosurgical practice. Much work is underway to develop *virtual reality* models of neurosurgical procedures with the aim of enabling trainees to acquire operative experience and to learn operative techniques without the need to 'practice' on patients [3]. The extensive range of technical manoeuvers and the variety of conditions met during a single operative procedure make this a daunting task. In theory, such computer based programmes could provide a method of assessment as well as training, but I suspect that we are many years away from using this as a feasible alternative.

Examination

After at least 4 years of clinical neurosurgical training in the UK, trainees sit an Intercollegiate Board Examination in Neurosurgery. This is comprised of two parts, the first, a MCQ on the applied neurosciences can be taken at any stage after appointment to a training programme. The second part is composed of a clinical exam of one hour duration, a 'spot' examination of one hour duration where slides of CT/MR images, histopathology, clinical features, operative anatomy etc. are shown to all candidates along with questions requiring short answers, and three $\times \frac{1}{2}$ hour vivas on 'operative surgery and surgical anatomy', 'the non-operative practice of neurosurgery', and' investigation of the neurosurgical patient'.

Such an examination tests clinical and basic scientific knowledge over a relatively wide range. The clinical and oral section tests history taking, patient examination, investigations, judgement and to a limited extent, communication, but time limitation restricts the range of topics. The examination does not evaluate decision-making, surgical skills and manual dexterity or experience; nor does it assess teaching, learning and management skills, personal effectiveness, or the ability to work in a team.

Other forms of examination such as the Objective Structured Clinical Examination (OSCE), consisting of short observations of clinical scenarios, utilising checklists to assess many clinical skills, can provide valid, reliable methods of testing many clinical skills, but these take considerable time and effort to develop and run [6].

Few other European countries conduct examinations in neurosurgery, but an examination of a similar standard is run by the European Association of Neurosurgical Societies (EANS). This EANS Board Examination is available in two parts. The first, an MCQ, is taken at any stage of training and the final part composed of three x 1 hour oral examinations, after completing one year in practice beyond gaining a CCST. Trainees from countries where no local examination exists should be encouraged to sit the EANS MCQ examination. Two countries have already made this a compulsory examination for their trainees.

Conclusions

Over the last 10 years in the United Kingdom and Ireland, we have established systematic procedures both locally and on a National level to evaluate trainees' progress throughout neurosurgical training. Present methods use a combination of in-training evaluation by the local trainers and the Training Programme Director, monitoring cumulative operative totals and an Intercollegiate examination. But operative totals reflect competence indirectly and could prove misleading. In-training evaluation by the trainers may give reliable information, particularly when multiple observers are involved [1], but at present this still lacks objectivity and validity. The suggested method of using competence tables or the structured technical skills assessment form may provide a useful addition to evaluating progress, but these still require validation in neurosurgical practice.

Despite the competitive selection process encountered before entering neurosurgical training, trainees progress at a variable rate. If it were feasible to measure clinical competence, then training could become "competence-based" rather than "time-based" – that is, the duration of training would depend on the time taken to achieve a certain level of competence rather than lasting a prescriptive minimum of 6 years. Whether or not these ideals are ever achieved, efforts to provide a more objective means of assessing competence can only improve current methods and raise the standards of training in general.

Appendix I. Joint committee on higher surgical training: trainee assessment form

This is an official document. A separate form is to be completed at the end of a placement by each trainer (forms are to be completed every 6 months and must be completed within a month of finishing the placement). The original is the property of the JCHST. Signed and completed forms are to be returned to the JCHST offices with a copy going to the Programme Director and Postgraduate Dean.

Guidance notes on the completion of this form are available on the JCHST web site, www.jchst.org from the Postgraduate Dean or Programme Director.

General Information

(to be completed in block capitals by trainee before handing to trainer for completion)

Form completed by (Name of trainer) ______________________________

Name of trainee ______________________________

Programme Director ______________________________

Specialty ______________________________

Training Number
(NTN/VTN/FTN or LAT) ______________________________

Expected CCST date (if applicable) ______________________________

GMC Number ______________________________

Post and Trust/Hospital
(Number if known) ______________________________

Assessment period From: ______________ To: ____________________

Sick Leave
Duration of absence due to sick leave during this period _______

Duration of sick leave since entering SpR training _______

Trainer Signature _________________________ Date____________________

Trainee Signature _________________________ Date____________________

September, 2001

To be completed by trainer

Year of SpR training (please circle) 6 mths 1 2 3 4 5 6

CRITERIA	unsatisfactory needs to repeat training in this area	needs targeted training in this area	satisfactory	COMMENTS
A. Clinical Skills				
History Taking				
Physical Exam				
Investigations				
Diagnosis				
Judgement				
Operative skill				
After care				

B Knowledge				
Basic Science				
Clinical				

C. Postgraduate Activities				
Teaching				
Lecturing				
Case presentation				
Publications				
Learning skills				
Research				
Audit				

CRITERIA	unsatisfactory needs to repeat training in this area	needs targeted training in this area	Satisfactory	COMMENTS
D. Attitudes				
Reliability				
Self Motivation				
Leadership				
Team working				
Administration				
Relationships & Communication With:				
a) Colleagues				
b) Patients				
c) Other staff				
Communication skills:-				
a) Informed consent				
b) Bereavement				
c) Breaking bad news				

Comments from trainer (please extend to an attached sheet if necessary – each attached sheet must be signed and dated by trainer and trainee)

____

____

____

____

____

____

____

Summary conclusion

❐ Satisfactory in all respects to proceed

❐ Satisfactory to proceed, but the following areas for improvement have been identified and must be addressed in the next placement (detail areas for improvement - please extend to an attached sheet if necessary –attached sheets must be signed and dated by trainer and trainee)

____

____

____

____

____

____

____

____

❐ Unsatisfactory to proceed and the training placement needs to be repeated

❐ Unsatisfactory and should be referred for advice to Postgraduate Dean / Programme Director about choosing an alternative career pathway

Comments from Trainee (please extend to an attached sheet if necessary – each attached sheet must be signed and dated by trainer and trainee)

____

____

____

____

____

____

____

____

Appendix II. Guidance notes on the completion of the JCHST Trainee Assessment form

1. The assessment form is CONFIDENTIAL once completed, and must be handled accordingly
2. Trainees are to complete the first section of the form **BEFORE** handing to their trainers.
3. It is a trainees responsibility to ensure that a separate form is completed by each of their consultant trainers
4. It is a trainees responsibility to ensure that a form (or forms) is completed at least every 6 months.
5. THE FORM WILL BE RETURNED IF INCOMPLETE

Assessors must take into account the year / level of training that the trainee has reached and assess accordingly.

Assessors are asked to put a X orin the appropriate column.

Assessors are to indicate any areas where improvements are necessary (requiring improvements does not necessarily mean a trainee will have to repeat training).

The columns below are not prescriptive but for guidance to how an assessment may differentiate between 'satisfactory' or 'in need of targeted training'. It is of overriding importance when completing this form and considering the performance of a trainee, that the trainee is judged in conjunction with the requirements of their specialty curriculum for their year of training and against the standards you would expect of their contemporaries. It is important that if deficiencies are identified these are evidence based and clearly noted.

Trainers are recommended to complete the form in draft PRIOR to meeting with the trainee.

CRITERIA	Examples of performance which would be considered unsatisfactory	Examples of performance which would be considered satisfactory
A. Clinical Skills		
History Taking	Incomplete, inaccurate. Poorly recorded	Complete, orderly, perceptive
Physical Exam	Misses important physical signs, relies unnecessarily on investigations	Thorough, accurate, can elicit correct signs, recognises most significant findings
Investigations	Inappropraite, random, inability to interpret tests	Usually appropriate, good knowledge on interpreting tests
Diagnosis	Fails to interpret and synthesise symptoms, signs and investigations	Good knowledge with an orderly logical approach to differential diagnosis, good clinical memory
Judgement	Difficulty in managing emergencies. Fails to take appropriate action	Reliable, competent under pressure, asks for advice appropriately
Operative skill	Not at competency level for year of training, treats tissues roughly, requires significant guidance	Competent to carry out procedures as required by the level of training
After care	Fails to notice complications and acts inappropriately	Good awareness of complications, takes appropriate action
B. Knowledge		
Basic Science	Not aware of the basic sciences applicable to the clinical practice	Adequate knowledge of the basic science related to the relevant surgical specialty
Clinical	Does not have necessary clinical knowledge	Adequate clinical knowledge to make decisions appropriate to year of training

CRITERIA	Examples of performance which would be considered unsatisfactory	Examples of performance which would be considered satisfactory
C. Postgraduate Activities		
Teaching	Appears uninterested in teaching. Contributes little to the education of juniors. Poor style.	Competent and conscientious in teaching others, good style
Lecturing	Inadequate preparation, poor style	A good speaker, well prepared and has prepared for questions
Case presentation	Needs to be better organised and/or better prepared. Poor on history, signs, diagnosis and discussion	History and signs correct, good deductions
Publications	Needs to complete writing up of a paper or thesis and to augment c.v. - no publications/presentations during period	Paper published or accepted for publication in a peer review journal or presentations at learned society during assessment period
Research	Not involved in research, poor graps of statistic and research methods	Able to critically analyse, involved in research and publishing results
Audit	Avoids audit, inadequare presentation	Involved in audit, good audit presentation
D. Attitudes		
Reliability	Poor time keeping, attention to detail and continuing patient care	Conscientious time keeper and in respect of patient care
Self Motivation	Disorganised in work practices, needing constant organisation and does not seek opportunities to learn	Able to organise working routine without supervision, looks for opportunities to learn
Leadership	Gives mixed and/or unclear instructions. Others not willing to be guided by the trainee	Gives clear instructions, able to motivate others. Setting a good example. Guide actions or opinions of others
Team working	Does not work well in a team: works alone and/or for own goals rather than team ones	Good relationships with team members, strive towards a common goal by co-operation and combined effort
Administration	Did not carry out the range of administrative duties required of post. Production of documentation not timely.	Carried out routine administration promptly and well. Has a good grasp of hospital management
Record Keeping	Inaccurate, insufficient information recorded, not timely, illegible	Accurate, inclusive and timely

Relationships & Communication with:

a) Colleagues	Poor rapport with both senior and junior colleagues: difficult to work with	Willing to help even if personally inconvenienced, able to defuse problems in the surgical team. Easy to work with
b) Patients	Does not establish a rapport, increases patients anxieties	Caring attitude. Listens well, explains well and can allay patients fears
c) Other Staff	Does not treat staff with respect. Is not approachable	Sound and professional yet approachable. Treats others with respect and is respected in return

Communication skills:

a) Informed consent	Gives inadequate details of procedures, risks and or alternatives. Is inappropriately persuasive	Able to obtain full informed consent, risks and alternatives explained clearly and well
b) Bereavement	Appears Casual: unfeeling	Sympathetic: empathetic
c) Breaking bad news	Inadequate explanations given: appears unsympathetic	Does in a sympathetic manner

The form is to be signed by trainer and trainee on completion

Appendix III. Confidential – joint committee on higher surgical training training post assessment form (for completion by higher surgical trainees)

This is an official document. The original is the property of the JCHST. After completion it should be passed to the Training Programme Director/Chair of the Regional Training Committee who will collate and scrutinise all reports relating to the programme, before making them available to the Regional Postgraduate Dean. The Training Programme Director/Chair of the Regional Training Committee will retain copies, submitting originals to the JCHST Office at The Royal College of Surgeons of England, 35/43 Lincoln's Inn Fields, London WC2A 3PE for scrutiny by the SACs.

TRAINEE NAME: .... **DATE:** ....

HOSPITAL BEING ASSESSED: .... **DATE STARTED:** ....

REGION: .... **NTN/VTN/FTN or LAT** ....

CONSULTANTS: .... **FROM:** .... **TO:** ....

SPECIALTY: .... **SPECIAL INTEREST(S):** ....

CLINICAL TRAINING	**Deficient**	**Satisfactory**	**Good**	**Comments**
Out Patients				
Special Clinics				
Ward Rounds				
Surgical Meeting				
Audit				
Journal Review				
OPERATIVE TEACHING				
Adequate Opportunity to Operate				
Demonstration of Techniques				
Supervision in Theatre				
Communication / Rapport with Consultant				
RESEARCH				
Opportunity				
(Detail Sessions............)				
Encouragement				
CAREER ADVICE				
CLINICAL MANAGEMENT				
1) Did the consultants allow adequate responsibility for patient management?				
2) Did you have adequate support with Emergency cases?				
a) in theatre				
b) advice				
FEEDBACK				
Did the Consultant provide you with appropriate feedback of your performance?				

GENERAL				

1) Strengths of firm: ______

2) Weaknesses of firm: ______

3) Suggestions for improvement: ______

4) Did this placement fulfil your expectations?

Deficient	Satisfactory	Good

OVERALL RATING

TRAINEE'S TIMETABLE

	Monday	Tuesday	Wednesday	Thursday	Friday	Saturday
Timetable (current)						

On Call – ROTA Tiers e.g. HST
ADH's SHO
PRHO

COURSES & MEETINGS ATTENDED IN LAST 12 MONTHS

Title	Date	Location

Number of days Study Leave granted ______

Course/meeting fee paid? **YES/NO**

Incidental expenses paid? **YES/NO**

These forms are strictly confidential. Completion and return will greatly facilitate the Department's activities.

NOTES TO ACCOMPANY JCHST TRAINING POST ASSESSMENT FORM

1. Assessment Form is **CONFIDENTIAL** once completed, and must be handled accordingly.
2. The following guidelines are for trainees completing the form.
   a. Complete as fully as possible the post details at the top of the form.
   b. Complete assessment by placing an 'X' in one box only against each criterion, with comments if desired. The following guidelines are offered for use in grading criteria.

	DEFICIENT	SATISFACTORY	GOOD
CLINICAL TRAINING			
Out patients	Do not see new patients. No time for / interest in discussion with consultant. Large number of patients. Poor organisation.	←→	See new & old patients. Time for discussion with consultant. Reasonable time with patient. Well organised.
Special Clinics	As above. Do not learn / use any special investigations / techniques. Often work alone.	←→	As above. Opportunity to learn special investigations / techniques. Often work with consultant. Multi disciplinary.
Ward Rounds	Rarely consultant led. Rapid decisions, little discussion. Junior views not listened to.	←→	Usually consultant led. In-depth presentation / discussion of patients. Adequate time allowed.
Surgical Meetings	Poor consultant support. Badly attended. Rigid non-innovative programme. Not multi-disciplinary. Held outside normal working hours. Little input from consultants.	←→	Consultant led. Well attended by all grades. Varied programme. Often multi-disciplinary. Regularly held in normal session time. Juniors encouraged to present / take part.
Audit	Morbidity / mortality only. No in-depth review of clinical practice / problems. Does not lead to change in clinical practice. Retrospective data. Juniors expected to collect all data. Non constructive / threatening atmosphere.	←→	Proper audit cycle utilised. Leads to change in clinical practice. Prospective data collection. Juniors assisted with data collection. Friendly, non-confrontational atmosphere.
Journal Review	Juniors expected to do all reviewing. Poor consultant attendance. Didactic discussion?	←→	Equal consultant / junior participation. Articles precied and discussed.
OPERATIVE TEACHING			
Opportunity	Usually left to do minor surgery. More than 5 elective sessions / week. Only assists and rarely performs more major cases.	←→	Mix of Major & minor elective surgery. At least 3 elective sessions / week. Exposure to day surgery, and minimal invasive surgery.

Teaching	Works on own. Poor senior support. Not shown / taught new or more advanced techniques.	↔	Taken through procedures. Shares cases with consultant. Video teaching films. Anastomotic and new technique workshops / courses encouraged.
Supervision	Consultant rarely present in same or adjoining theatre. Own lists. Cannot readily summon senior assistance if in difficulty. No clear guidelines.	↔	Consultant usually present in same or adjoining theatre. Assistance at senior level readily available. Given clear guidelines as to when to call / inform / discuss with consultant.
RESEARCH			
Opportunity	No fixed time allowed. Any identified time often not taken due to other pressures. Clinical work precludes time for research.	↔	Fixed session / protected time allocated. Arrangements made to free trainee of some clinical work to allow research activity.
Encouragement	No interest shown by consultants. No ideas or stimulation.	↔	Able to discuss / plan ideas with consultants. Directed to appropriate sources for information / opportunities / funding.
CAREER ADVICE			
	Consultant not interested in trainee or his career.	↔	Consultant offers advice / help. Directs trainee to source of advice / help.
CLINICAL MANAGEMENT			
Patient Management	No guidelines. No trust. Consultant questions all decisions. Consultant does not back trainee.	↔	Consultant readily offers help / advice. Trainee given guidelines. Trusted to use own initiative / judgement. Consultant backs trainee.
Emergency Operating	Advice / help not easy to obtain. Consultant difficult to find / contact. Also not keen to come in / assist.	↔	Advice / help readily available. Consultant always happy to be phoned / consulted / give advice.
Feedback	Poor or absent appraisal. No specified protected time for discussion of trainee's performance. Consultant not frank about performance. Mainly critical. Rarely praises.	↔	Regular appraisals sessions in clearly specified time. Consultants open about strengths / weaknesses / areas for improvement.
GENERAL			
	No objectives. All clinical work. Poor education / learning.	↔	Clear objectives for trainee. Good balance / clinical / teaching / learning / research.

References

1. CanMeds 2000 Project. Skills for the new millennium: report of the social needs working group. Sept. 1996. Royal College of Physicians and Surgeons of Canada
2. Darzi A, Smith S, Taffinder N (1999) Assessing operative skill. *Brit Med J* 318: 888–889
3. Haase J, Musaeus P, Boisen E (2001) Virtual reality and habitats for learning microsurgical skills. (in press)
4. Lindsay K.W (2002) Neurosurgical training in the UK and Ireland: assessing progress and attainment. *Neurosurgery.* 50: 1103–1113
5. Martin JA, Regehr G, Reznick RK *et al* (1997) Objective structural assessment of technical skill (OSAT) for surgical residents. Br J Surg 84: 273–278
6. Merrick HW, Nowacek GA, Padgett B, Francis B, Gohara SF, Staren ED (2002) Ability of the objective structured clinical examination to differentiate surgical residents, medical students, and physician assistant students. *J Surg Res* 106: 319–322
7. Reznick RK, Regehr G, Martin J *et al* (1997) Testing technical skills via an innovative 'Bench Station' examination. *Am J Surg* 173: 226–230
8. Richards R (1999) Why do we need to assess competence? In *Surgical Competence.* Royal College of Surgeons of England, London, pp 6–15
9. Winckel CP, Reznick RK, Cohen R, Taylor B (1994) Reliability and construct validity of a structured technical skills assessment form. *Am J Surg* 167: 423–427.

Correspondence: K. W. Lindsay, Department of Neurosurgery, Southern General Hospital, Govan Road, Glasgow G51 4TF, UK. e-mail: kwlindsay@sgh.scot.nhs.uk

Acta Neurochir (2004) [Suppl] 90: 97–101

Printed in Austria

XII Research rotation in a trainee's curriculum

H.-J. Reulen[1] and **Y. Kanpolat**[2]

[1] Department of Neurosurgery, Ludwig-Maximilians-University, Klinikum Großhadern, Munich, Germany
[2] Yücel Kanpolat, Neurosurgical Department, Ankara University, Turkey

Introduction

All over the world, residency programmes for neurosurgery emphasize heavily technical issues. This training, more or less successful, teaches surgical techniques and procedures to neurosurgery trainees. Other issues, for instance training of administrative capabilities, despite their obvious importance in the life of a neurosurgeon, do not receive the merit they deserve. Research constitutes another important element in the training programme. For some, research is a matter of science to be conducted only by academicians in centers of quality. However, research, as a key component of occupational practice and indeed of life in general, should be stressed. This article aims at discussing the role and methods of application of research within neurosurgical practice.

The goals of a research rotation

What do we expect and what are the goals of a research rotation? Most of the academic programme directors or chairmen consider a research period an essential component of education, although most agree that not every resident needs such a rotation [4, 5, 7, 10, 12, 13, 14, 15, 16]. If we look at the background of our successful neurosurgical teachers, most of them had such an elective exposure to research. The goal of a well-organized research rotation is to gain an understanding of the intellectual processes involved in collecting, analyzing and interpreting clinical observations in a systematic way [1, 2, 8, 9]. Such experience will significantly improve the individual's rational approach to the management of patients, and the critical judgment of his own work and, for instance, the literature [10], when later he works outside a clinical environment.

George Ojeman in 1985 [10, 11] wrote about the role of research training in a neurosurgical residency: "The essential features of research are making systematic observations and organizing these into hypothesis and written documents. Often, but not always, this is done in a planned experiment. With this general definition, research training has a place in every neurosurgical residency programme regardless of the trainee's ultimate career goals and even if they do not continue with research, for opportunities to make new observations – of unique cases, the effects of therapy, pathophysiology of neurosurgical diseases, or the function of the nervous system- will occur in every neurosurgical career."

Additional goals could be added which may represent a second level. The resident should be introduced to the art of science in a way that he learns and experiences the real excitement of uncovering and describing new knowledge. Also he should come to a point where he is able to start his own research project, raise funds, and teach students and younger colleagues.

It is a matter of fact that in our training institutions there are residents who are planning an academic career, and others who plan to practise, although it must be stressed that many trainees at the early stage of their careers are unsure of their interests. With the above definitions a wide range of options can be offered to both groups, according to their specific interests.

Structures and categories of research

Different structures are used to organize research rotations. Some departments focus exclusively on re-

Table 1. *Categories of Research in Neurosurgery*

A.	Fundamental basic neurosciences (blue sky research)
B.	Laboratory studies simulating clinical diseases (experimental cerebral vasospasm, brain edema, experimental brain tumors, etc.)
C.	Applied clinical research (application of basic research techniques to a clinical problem)
D.	Research related to technical innovations and to improving surgical techniques (neuronavigation, functional mapping, laser-teachnique, instrumentation and biomechanics)
E.	Clinical observational studies (restrospective studies, case reports, prospective non-randomized studies, studies on natural course or outcome)
F.	Randomized prospective controlled trials

search training in a laboratory within the department under the guidance of neurosurgical faculty members experienced in research. Others prefer to send their trainees to a different institution where applied clinical research is performed, particularly if the department in question does not have appropriate conditions, and finally a third group of departments prefer rotation in an area of basic research in one of the basic neuroscience institutions. Thus, as shown in Table 1, a wide range of possibilities exists today, extending from fundamental basic research in neurosciences to patient-oriented studies and finally to randomized controlled trials (Table 1).

The important question is whether all these options do have the same rating in the context of neurosurgical training. Can we achieve the above-defined goals of research both with a rotation in basic research for instance tissue slices- or by participating in a prospective clinical trial?

Selection of a research area

There are certainly arguments that strongly support clinically oriented research. This is advocated by most of the experienced programme directors. A successful academic career depends on two columns: a) performance of competent clinical patient care and b) generation of high-level research [15]. Thus clinical practice and research projects regularly compete for the academic neurosurgeon's time, particularly if other tasks like administration, teaching, etc. have also to be performed. In contrast to colleagues in neurology or internal medicine, surgeons spend a large part of their day in the operating theater. The time remaining for research projects is always limited. Therefore when choosing a research area, there are definite advantages of combining research with the individual's field of clinical interest, for instance working on vasospasm if the main clinical interest is vascular neurosurgery. Thus the neurosurgeon may use questions posed on a ward round as subject for an adequate study, be it experimental or clinical. Such studies are likely to influence the neurosurgeon's future practice.

During the past 25 years a deep shift in the understanding and execution of neurosurgery has occurred. Between 1960 and 1970, it was still possible for one person to have an overview of more or less all technical procedures as well as the theoretical knowledge. Most of the scientific neurosurgical publications at that time were understandable and of interest to the majority of neurosurgeons.

In the last 10 to 15 years neurosurgeons have tried to increasingly concentrate on specific areas as for instance neurooncology, functional and stereotactic surgery, spinal neurosurgery, skull base surgery, posterior fossa surgery, pediatric neurosurgery, etc. and consequently in all those fields a more profound knowledge has built up involving new technical operative skills and procedures, and improvement of the technical tools, etc. This finally led to the development of subspecialty areas as seen today in many departments, a development which offers to patients a higher competence in a specific section and which cannot be reversed. In any of those subspecialties the literature has increased considerably so that today it has become impossible to comprehend or even obtain all the new information. Furthermore a growing inclination can be observed to plan and organize research projects in a way that the criteria for class I evidence are met [8, 15].

This change in paradigm coincided with a change in fields of research. There are now many more research areas than in the 60s or 70s. Each one of the subspecialty areas comprises many responsibilities, again ranging from basic research to randomized controlled clinical trials, as shown in Table 1.

As a consequence and taking into account the obvious tendency of our young colleagues to focus their clinical work on one of the various subspecialty areas of neurosurgery, the choice of the research topic will become even more important. Two examples are given below:

a) A resident in his/her third or fourth year of training received a fairly good overview of most clinical areas. The resident decides that his/her major interest is spinal neurosurgery, and, after finishing his/her regular training programme, wishes to acquire special knowledge in this field by entering a respective fellowship in spinal neurosurgery. It would be logical to choose as research rotation a project closely related to the resident's future work, in this case for instance spinal neuronavigation, spinal surgical anatomy, spinal biomechanics, or instrumentation, etc.

It would not be logical or even a waste of time, however, if this resident got involved for example in studies on hippocampus slices, in experimental studies on vasospasm, or in any other project remote from his/her clinical interest. Even with the best introduction into the art of science, the final result of such studies would not likely substantially influence his/her practice in spinal neurosurgery. It is most probable that at the end of such a research rotation, the resident would drop these studies. Such a wrong selection of research is one of the reasons why many young neurosurgeons after years of research and successful publications do not pursue their activities after having received their PhD or title of professor. This is obviously a waste, as such well educated colleagues would rather be qualified to instruct younger trainees. The interest of the trainees should be taken into consideration.

b) Another trainee at the end of his/her second or third year of training sees his/her future commitment in neurooncology and plans to add a neurooncological fellowship after having finished the regular residency programme. After several talks with the programme director the resident uses his/her elective time to work 6 months in an oncology department to learn the theoretical and practical principles of chemotherapy and then participates as the local investigator in a multicenter prospective randomized study on brain tumor therapy. There is no doubt that with appropriate supervision and support, this trainee will learn much from such an experience. With this knowledge the resident will be able to later extend his/her studies and organize projects independently. The authors are convinced that it is one of the important goals of training that at a certain point our trainees become independent and able to organize their own research projects. Such candidates will form the future cadres in academic neurosurgery and also represent the necessary links to the other neuroscience communities [8].

In planning the neurosurgical training programme, when should research begin?

Should it be done at the beginning or even before starting clinical practice, after a certain time of clinical exposure or rather towards the end of the programme?

Probably there is no definite and generally valid answer to this question since one will find individual success stories for all three situations. However, there are convincing arguments that a research rotation should be recommended for the majority of our trainees after at least one, but not later than three or four years of clinical practice in neurosurgery [11]. It seems wise to first observe the clinical abilities and conduct of a young trainee, and then, only in cooperation with him, choose a suitable scientific activity.

The other extreme would be to organize the research period at the end of the residency programme. At that stage, an intelligent resident would know his/her clinical interests and also have the desire to acquire the tools for a more systematic and scientific approach to some unsolved problems. However, this is exactly the time when surgical progress and success are greatest and the resident's interests are focused entirely on improving his/her surgical skills and techniques, and acquiring new surgical methods, etc. There will certainly be a collision of interests. Oftentimes this conflict is resolved based on economic restraints, and in the process some very gifted young colleagues are lost.

If the resident starts with a period of clinical neurosurgery, there are obvious advantages for both teacher and trainee. The arguments for the teacher are: The resident can be observed in his/her clinical and social performance, problem-solving skills, ability to perform under stress, manual dexterity, judgment, etc. The teacher can obtain an idea of his/her talents through observation and regular evaluation by the staff members. He can discuss with the resident his/her abilities and interests and find the best solution for this individual. It should be attempted to define a research area that motivates the trainee for a long time and thus lead to success! The candidate has time to look for a suitable research position in his own or in another department or in another institution. The chosen position should serve the interests of both the resident and those of the department, if one considers eventually a continuing activity in a research project. Hence selection of the topic and of the laboratory is a very important task! It is of no benefit to have the resident participating only as a technician in an ongoing project, he/she should be provided with the skill for independent research and the time to prepare funding of a research rotation, if necessary.

Vice versa, during this initial clinical period, the resident has the chance to examine whether or not his decision for neurosurgery as a career was the right one. He will find out how genuine his commitment to patient management really is and pursue training with more passionate intensity. He learns to deal with the unusual, complex case where he sees that routine alone is not sufficient and that search of literature and reading become necessary. He has the opportunity to observe the work of various specialists and to develop a specific interest, for instance in vascular or spinal problems, etc. With this background he can plan his research rotation more specifically, and may have an opportunity to participate in a research project.

The role of the programme director

From the previous discussion it results that the chairman, the programme director or an assigned tutor has high responsibility in advising the trainee in the above-described decision process and in preparing a research rotation. It is important that the trainee's abilities and interests are discussed with him/her at regular intervals. As soon as the trainee has developed a specific preference for one of the various subspecialty areas, a suitable research topic should be defined. Selection of the research project should be tailored to the individual trainee's clinical interests. The next step would be to choose a well-suited laboratory or another department to best serve the needs of the resident for his research rotation. The staff member in such a system certainly plays an important role in the career planning of the resident [4, 7, 11]. Such a procedure will enhance the success of a research rotation and chances that the trainee will later continue research as part of his career. Furthermore, the rotational proceeding will no doubt prefer clinically oriented research and reduce purely basic research, as defined previously.

Outlook

Today it is knowledge, the product of human intellect, that drives modern society. Knowledge in the form of scientific achievement, know-how and technology are the commodities worth the greatest value. Scientific achievement controls the industry, agriculture, health and the environment as well as all the other important lifelines of modern living [16].

Modern society will flourish from knowledge that is the product of scientific research. Research is not only individual scientific action carried out by small groups of scientists, on subjects that are of interest to their narrow involvement, but also a component of a general concerted scientific action that is launched for the purpose of creating a science-based, science-driven society, to serve sustainable economic competitiveness of nations and the future welfare of their people.

In this vein, the European Community has completed the fifth of such programmes, termed Framework Programmes (FP), focused on raising scientific research capability and quality of the European society. The sixth such programme was initiated in 2002 [3]. The 17.5 billion EURO FP6 will allocate as much as 10.5 billion EURO (about 62%) to the European Research Area (ERA) projects that consist of funding research in 7 fields considered of vital importance in building the future of the European society, based on science and technology [3]. Europe is another such programme that envisages building an information society allowing easy and wide access to information and automation of official applications and technicalities.

Conclusions

Research rotation is an important component in the education of a neurosurgical trainee.

Selection of research should be tailored to the individual trainee's clinical interest.

Avoid studies remote from the individual trainee's clinical interest.

Select a proper laboratory, institution or clinical research programme for the research rotation.

If possible utilize the advantages of cooperation with other institutions.

References

1. Baethmann A, Messmer K (1992) Stellung der klinischen Forschung in der Chirurgie: Konzept der Experimentellen Chirurgie. Chirurg BDC 31 [Suppl] 1: 29–33
2. Baethmann A, Meßmer K (1992) Experimentelle Chirurgie. In: Schweiberer L, Izebicki IR (eds) Akademische Chirurgie. Springer, Berlin Heidelberg New York Tokyo, pp 177–181
3. Commission of the European Union, Communication to the European Parliament concerning the common position of the Council about the 6th Framework Programme of the European Community for research, technological development and dem-

onstration activities contributing to the creation of the European Research Area (2002–2006) and to innovation – 30.01.02
4. Fahlbusch R (1997) From the scientific idea to its realisation. Principles and Strategies in Neurosurgery. Acta Neurochir (Wien) [Suppl] 69: 120–125
5. Hoff JT (1994) Toward better balance. The 1994 presidential address. J Neurosurg 81: 651–655
6. Kanpolat Y (2002) Significance of research, research and publishing in neurosurgery. In: Kanpolat Y (ed) Acta Neurochir (Wien) [Suppl] 83: 1–5
7. Langfitt Th W (1982) Research and training in the neurosurgical sciences, J Neurosurg 57: 733–738
8. Messmer K, Baethmann A (1997) Role of surgical research in the training of neurosurgeons. Acta Neurochir (Wien) [Suppl] 69: 111–115
9. Messmer K (1990) Perspektiven der Experimentellen Chirurgie. Chirurg 61: 248–250
10. Ojeman GA (1985) The role of research rotation in a neurosurgical residency. Neurosurgery 17: 138–139
11. Ojemann RG (1992) Training the neurosurgeon for the twenty-first century. Surg Neurol 37: 167–174
12. Pickard JD. (1995) What is neurosurgical research? Acta Neurochir (Wien) 133: 236–238
13. Reulen HJ, Olteanu-Nerbe V, Steiger HJ (1996) The neurosurgical clinic at the Ludwig-Maximilians-University in Munich. Neurosurgery 39: 1224–1231
14. Reulen HJ (1997) When should residents be exposed to research Acta Neurochir (Wien) [Suppl] 69: 106–110
15. Teasdale GM (1997) Research in Neurosurgical Training. Clinical reviews and trials. Acta Neurochir (Wien) [Suppl] 69: 116–119
16. Yoshimoto T, Tominaga T (1997) Contents and structure of a training rogramme. The Japanese proposal. Acta Neurochir (Wien) [Suppl] 69: 81–83

Correspondence: Prof. Dr. H.-J. Reulen, Schwojer Str. 19, 81249 Munich, Germany. e-mail: Ilona.Anders@med.uni-muenchen

Acta Neurochir (2004) [Suppl] 90: 103–106

Printed in Austria

XIII The accreditation of a training programme

H.-J. Reulen

Department of Neurosurgery, Ludwig-Maximilians-University, Klinikum Großhadern, Munich, Germany

General information

The U.E.M.S. has been active in the field of quality improvement of specialist training in the EU for years and has formulated general guidelines and criteria, published in the European Training Charter for Medical Specialists [1]. In accordance with these guidelines, the UEMS specialist sections develop specific recommendations to set and maintain standards of training, training quality and accreditation of training institutions for the respective speciality. Also they should monitor the contents and the quality of training. This aids harmonization of the training level in the EC. At a national level, training of medical specialists is regulated by the national authorities [1] who set standards in accordance with their national rules and EC legislation as well as in consideration of the UEMS/European Board recommendations.

An important feed-back instrumentation for quality improvement is the visitation and evaluation of training centers, which in future may be coupled with certification and recertification of trainers. At present an external evaluation of the quality of training exists in only a few of the countries of the EU, and the national approaches differ considerably. Therefore, in the UEMS, the need was felt for a harmonisation and encouragement in the field of visitation of training centers. The new *European Charter on Visitation of Training Centers*, 2002 [3] presents the outlines as to organize a national programme for visitation of training centers. The following definitions are made by the UEMS.

Statutory visitation

The responsible national authority is recommended to establish programmes for this purpose as far as these have not been developed yet. Such programmes are increasingly required and tend to become obligatory, as is already the case in several member states of the EU.

Voluntary visitation

Training centers are encouraged to participate in voluntary visitation programmes that award additional quality titles. The UEMS European Boards are active in this field [3].

In Neurosurgery the EANS and the Section of Neurosurgery of the UEMS have entrusted the *Joint Residency Advisory and Accreditation Committee (JRAAC)* with the above task, i.e. the preparatory work for the visitation of European neurosurgical training centres. The visitation programme is now being offered on a voluntary basis for a European recognition of quality of teaching and training in Neurosurgery by the JRAAC. Training centers in Europe are encouraged to participate in such a voluntary visitation programme. Since this European visitation programme follows the highest standards, it should be secured that in the future an accreditation issued by JRAAC as an UEMS/EANS body is recognized by the national authorities.

In the following it is described how the European Accreditation of a Training Programme is organized.

The application

a) The Programme Director must submit the *Programme Application Form* to the Secretary of the JRAAC to arrive sufficiently in advance of a Committee Meeting to allow for proper reviewing. In future a second questionnaire will have to be completed by a representative of the trainees. Applications will be evaluated within the subsequent 6 months. The Programme Application Form can be obtained from the Chairman or the Secretary of JRAAC (presently Prof. T. Trojanowski or Prof. M. Zerah, secretary) or be downloaded from the website of the EANS (www.eans.org/→committees →accreditation form).

b) The Application Form has to be completed in detail by the applying department, describing the personnel, space, technical facilities, clinical experience available, and in particular their Residency Training Programme. The data are necessary for the Evaluation Committee to assess the status of the Residency Programme. The completed Application Form should be sent to one of the addresses given below (see Important addresses).

c) The completed Programme Application Form will be reviewed by at least two members of the JRAAC. The reviewers may request additional material directly from the Programme Director and shall prepare a proposal for the next JRAAC committee meeting.

The site visit

a) If the Training Programme according to the Application Form is in essential compliance with the requirements, the next step will be a *Site Visit* of the applying institution, conducted by two independent visitors (experienced chairpersons) nominated by the JRAAC, and a third national observer/visitor appointed by the applying institution. One member will act as Chairman, another as secretary. The national visitor acts as an observer, may help explain national requirements and peculiarities and should be an experienced member of the respective National Neurosurgical Society. The date of the Site Visit will be arranged between the Programme Director and the site visitors as soon as possible. The Programme Director will receive the necessary information to prepare the time table of the site visit in due time. The site visit will be performed according to the Guidelines of the UEMS Charter on Visitation of Training Centers (2002) [3]. The Site Visit preferably lasts 1 day and serves to see the hospital(s) and department(s) involved in the Training Programme and the educational and scientific environment, holding personal discussions with the Programme Director, the Chairman, the teachers, the trainees, and a representative of the administration. A team discussion with the trainees may be helpful as well. Information given by the trainees must remain confidential. Concluding the visit, a debate with the teaching staff should take place. The time table should include a 30 minute section for the visiting team to formulate its conclusions, conditions and recommendations. Details can be added later when a report is compiled. The center being visited is responsible for the expenses of travel and local accommodation of the site visitors.

A *report* will be prepared by the site visitors for the subsequent meeting of the JRAAC. The training center should be granted an inspection of the draft of the report to correct any factual errors. The final report will be part of the final decision on the accreditation status of the Programme. Confidentiality regarding the contents of the site visitors' report must strictly be adhered to by the site visitors. All information obtained during the interviews with trainers and trainees remain absolutely confidential.

b) The *accreditation status* as decided by the JRAAC will be reported to the respective Programme Director by formal Letter of Notification. The letter will be forwarded by the Committee Chairman within a reasonable period of time following the committee meeting. On request of the Programme Director, the Dean of the Faculty and/or authorities of the hospital also may receive the official report. Together with the report additional advice and recommendations if necessary will be given to further improve the Training Programme.

The accreditation

The following decisions may be taken by the JRAAC with regard to the accreditation status of a Training Institution and Programme.

Full accreditation (accreditation at full status) may be granted by the JRAAC if the programme has demonstrated to be in full compliance with the Essentials of the European Training Charter [1], the Essentials to Organize a Residency Training Programme [2], and the Charter on Visitation of Training Centers [3]. The Department that has been fully accredited will receive a certificate indicating that the Department and the

Residency Programme fulfil the criteria to meet European Standards of Excellence for Education in Neurosurgery. The certificate is issued by the Chairman and the Secretary of the JRAAC and co-signed by the President of the Section of Neurosurgery of the U.E.M.S. as well as the President of EANS. The accreditation shall be re-assessed after 5 years or within one year after change of a Programme Director.

Provisional accreditation indicates that the programme is basically in line (not in compliance) with the above cited requirements and standards. It is considered as being in a status of development. The Programme Director will be requested to submit a so-called *Progress Report* within one or two years after notification. The Committee shall exactly specify the information to be provided. When a Progress Report is asked for, a specific due date should be included in the request.

Accreditation may be withheld if the programme does not substantially comply with the essentials of the above defined requirements and standards. The Committee will cite those areas in which the reviewed programme does not comply with the standards. A new application can be submitted when the areas indicated are brought in compliance with the requirements and standards.

Accreditation may be discontinued if a programme for some reason is no longer in compliance with the requirements and standards defined above. A new application can be submitted if the requirements are again fulfilled.

Reassessment of a Programme is usually done after 5 years or within one year after change of a Programme Director. For re-assessment the Application Form must be supplemented with the desired data of the calendar year before.

Confidentiality

Information as well as documents acquired during the accreditation process (application form, site visit report) as well as the decisions of the JRAAC remain strictly confidential. The training center that has been visited is entitled to make public the visitation report and the certification. JRAAC will publish the following information about accredited programmes in Acta Neurochirurgica: name and address of the training center, name of the programme director.

Commentary

Some comments shall be made on the present status of the external evaluation and accreditation process.

Experiences gathered so far by the members of JRAAC with regard to the evaluation of a number of departments have shown some interesting aspects: In various European countries individual departments, national neurosurgical societies, or national authorities to some extent have previously developed some form of local or national log-book, an educational programme, etc.; i.e. they established their own requirements and standards for the training of their residents, set up of course in their national language. This made judgement sometimes very difficult for the Review Committee members and thus the role of the national observer during the site visit became very important in explaining the respective background or translating some of the important written material. This diversity at present is typical for the European situation and is taken into account by the JRAAC when making their decision concerning the accreditation status. On the other side it has been observed – although the training programmes of the visited departments generally were on a good or high level – that several "deficits" existed in most of the training centers regarding the formal organisation of a programme in general, the periodic internal progress assessment, the involvement of the resident in all areas of our specialty, and in particular the rotations. The Programme Directors of the visited departments, therefore, received together with the Accreditation of the Training Programme a detailed report specifying those areas where the Review Committee thought were deficits. In addition, a *Progress Report* was asked for after one or two years to show how such deficiencies have been improved.

The Charter on Training of Specialists in the EC and particularly the requirements and standards defined by the UEMS Section of Neurosurgery have been in existence for a few years only and therefore "full compliance" with all the requirements at this time cannot be expected. The new edition of the Charter on Training is being written in summer and fall of 2003 and will probably be available in 2004. It defines more precisely the requirements for a training center as well as the contents of a training programme and thus facilitates their implementation in practice. The national societies or the responsible authorities in a country will now have the responsibility to adapt their requirements and criteria to the UEMS/European Board recommendations. This certainly will lead to a further harmonization of the training in our speciality. At present we still have the great chance of being able to define our standards ourselves, but we have to seize this unique opportunity.

The staff groups of the centers visited so far all expressed that the whole evaluation process, the preparation of the Application Form, the site visit, and the report represented a very positive experience. During the compilation of the extensive material for the Application Form, a new insight into the organisation, the working processes, the strengths and weaknesses etc. of the department could be gained. During the evaluation process and particularly the site visit, they receive friendly advice and support from a group of experienced colleagues in order to complete or upgrade their programmes to be in compliance with the new European standards. Also the trainees regarded the exchange with the site visitors as helpful and they were proud to pass their training in an institution with a quality mark of the EANS and UEMS. With very high probability, intelligent and gifted young colleagues who want to apply for a training position will in future give their preference to institutions with such a quality mark.

Proposal of a time table for visitation

There should be a preliminary meeting (working dinner) with the Chairman, staff members, and the visitation team the evening before the visitation.

The general frame of the department, its collaboration with neighbouring specialities, advantages and deficits can be discussed. Also a general outline of the training programme or specific national requirements may be given.

These are the main sites of interest for the site visitors. Others may be given in the letter to the Programme Director.

Time table (Example)

.... morning conference

.... conference with all staff members

visit of the department

- operating theatre
- intensive care
- outpatient department
- general ward
- neuroradiology/imaging, endovascular techniques,
- radiotherapy or radiosurgery as available
- library and computer facilities
- research facilities
- records

.... interview with trainees (individual and confidential)

.... (the trainees should have their Log-Book available)

.... interview with Medical Director and/or Administrative Director

.... discussion with Chairman and/or Programme Director summary

.... concluding session for the visiting team (30 mins)

References

1. European Training Charter (Charter on Training of Medical Specialists in the EC) U.E.M.S., Secretariat Avenue de al Couronne 20, B – Bruxelles, 1995 – www.uems.be/5charte.htm
2. "Essentials to organize a Residency Training Programme". (1998) Acta Neurochir (Wien) 141: 731–733
3. Charter on Visitation of Training Centres (U.E.M.S., 24 October 1997) – www.uems.be/visitati.htm

Correspondence: Prof. Dr. H.-J. Reulen, Schwojer Str. 19, 81249 Munich, Germany. e-mail: Ilona.Anders@med.uni-muenchen.de

Acta Neurochir (2004) [Suppl] 90: 107–114

Printed in Austria

XIV The European Examination – its present status and potential development

J. Haase

Department of Health Science and Technology, Aalborg University, Aalborg, Denmark

Too much knowledge leads to over activity;
Better to calm the mind.
The more you consider, the greater the loss;
Better to unify the mind
Excessive thinking weakens the will.
The more you know, the more your mind is confused;
A confused mind gives rise to vexation.
Merely reading books is of no lasting value
(Wang Ming)

Historical background

The diversity among the over 30 European countries sending trainees to the EANS training courses is immense. This is based on both cultural factors and differences in priorities of teaching in the different countries. The explosion of medical knowledge poses an additional challenge to all those responsible in setting priorities for what is thought to be the core knowledge in a given training programme. With the concept of developing European standards in neurosurgical training it was evident that an evaluation of both trainers and trainees was necessary. In the US, already in 1940 the first American Board of Neurological Surgeons (ABNS) examination took place. In the UK, the first Intercollegiate Specialty Board Examination was held in 1991, consisting of a multiple-choice questionnaire (MCQ), a clinical examination and 3 vivas [13]. The objective of such examinations is to assure a certain level of theoretical and practical knowledge and to establish safety. While the majority of chairmen believe that such a set of exams is the best available method for probing clinical judgment and knowledge regarding the management of patients, others express a more critical view as for instance stated by John Picard: "Certainly my personal impression, unsubstantiated by any official statistics, is that the level of excellence in the examination does not correlate with subsequent progress, academic innovation, or medical legal complications [13]."

Within the EANS, Mario Brock and Reinder Braakman [5] stimulated the creation of a committee with the aim to develop a European examination of a similar standard as those described above. In 1991, this committee published the recommendations and plans: "Towards a European Board of Neurological Surgery" [5] which was accepted by the EANS Administrative Council. The Examination Committee of the EANS was then founded, chaired by Reinder Braakman. He and subsequently Hans-J. Reulen and Jens Haase were invited guests of the American Board of Neurological Surgeons (ABNS) both at their multiple choice exam (MCQ) and at the oral examinations, and these visits implemented important information in our own EANS setup. Instead of long fruitless discussions on the validity of testing, the European Exam was finally constructed using established features of the ABNS – trying to give all trainees a platform of minimal requirements for being a practicing neurosurgeon in Europe.

The exam was designed with a primary Multiple Choice exam (MCQ) on different main topics and a final oral exam after a trainee had received his/her authorization as a neurosurgeon and having been practicing for 2 years

The updated **guidelines** of the European Exam can be found in addendum 1.

Primary Multiple Choice Examination (MCQ)

In 1992 the first MCQ exam was held with 57 trainees and a passing rate of 33%. After the initial testing of the system, the MCQ exam in 1994 in Turkey attracted 64 participants, the largest number ever! The drop of participants to 34 in 1996 and later down to a mere 12 was unacceptable with regard to the basic ideas of the exam. This led to a critical re-evaluation within the Examination Committee and the Administrative Council (AC) of the EANS. A breakthrough occurred when the Swiss and later the Swedish neurosurgical societies decided to have the MCQ as an integral part of their national specialization in neurosurgery. It was suggested in the AC that this should be extended to all European nations. Finally in 2001, the AC of the EANS decided to make the MCQ an integral part of the EANS Courses with the given consent of the trainees. Since then all 4th and 5th year trainees are taking the MCQ during the last course of their cycle at no cost.

The Examination Committee selects from a pool of questions in various categories around 180 questions for each exam. The pool consists of new and old questions kept strictly confidential.

The questions are prepared by the appointed committee according to the following guidelines: use of simple, "European English" language, with 5 possible answers of which one is correct, possible answers always in alphabetical order.

An example is shown in Table 1.

Table 1.

x) Plateau waves (type A waves of Lundberg)
a: are related to periodic breathing
b: have a low amplitude
c: have no clinical significance
*d: indicate reduced craniospinal compliance
e: usually last less than one minute

The answers are approximately of the same length. The only correct answer is marked with *.

Questions where e.g. 2 out of 5 answers may be correct, as used elsewhere, have not been included so far.

Another set of questions was later introduced being of a yes/no type, an example of which is given in Table 2.

Table 2.

y) The formation rate of cerebrospinal fluid in congenital hydrocephalus is normal
*a: true
b: false

The correct answer is also marked with *.

All previous and newly structured questions are evaluated by an MCQ expert to secure answer quality statistically. A question should not be too simple and provide nearly 100% correct answers, nor should it allow more than one correct answer. Such answers are removed from the question pool.

The exam is taken during a 3-hour-period in two parts, A and B with a short intermission. The trainees cannot remove the original question sheets from the examination room. We have emphasized that cheating during the exam will result in direct demission but have never seen any example of this. Each trainee receives his/her personal results and evaluations together with the average result of the whole group in order to visualize weak points.

An example of the gross evaluation of the 2002 exam is shown in Table 3.

Table 3 presents an overview of the primary exam of August 2002. In part A of the exam 5 questions were found to be invalid and therefore were removed from

Table 3. *European Association of Neurosurgical Societies. European Primary Examination, August, 2002*

Final Result	
Total Examination Valid Questions = 174 of 180 Participants = 46 Sum of Scores = 4693 Mean Score = 102.02 (58.63%) Standard deviation = 18.56	
Neuroanatomy	(17 Questions): 10.76 (63.30%)
Neuropathophysiology	(20 Questions): 11.61 (58.04%)
Neurology	(14 Questions): 8.28 (59.16%)
General skills	(10 Questions): 5.50 (55.00%)
Head Injury	(7 Questions): 3.48 (49.69%)
Brain Tumours	(29 Questions): 17.26 (59.52%)
Cerebrovascular Disease	(30 Questions): 16.72 (55.72%)
Peripheral Nerves	(10 Questions): 6.07 (60.65%)
Spine and Cord	(24 Questions): 13.57 (56.52%)
Neuroradiology	(3 Questions): 2.63 (87.68%)
Pediatric and Congential	(10 Questions): 6.15 (61.52%)
Part A Valid Questions = 90 of 95 Participants = 46 Sum of Scores = 2457 Mean Score = 53.41 (59.35%) Standard deviation = 11.54	
Part B Valid Questions = 84 of 85 Participants = 46 Sum of Scores = 2236 Mean Score = 48.61 (57.87%) Standard deviation = 7.95	

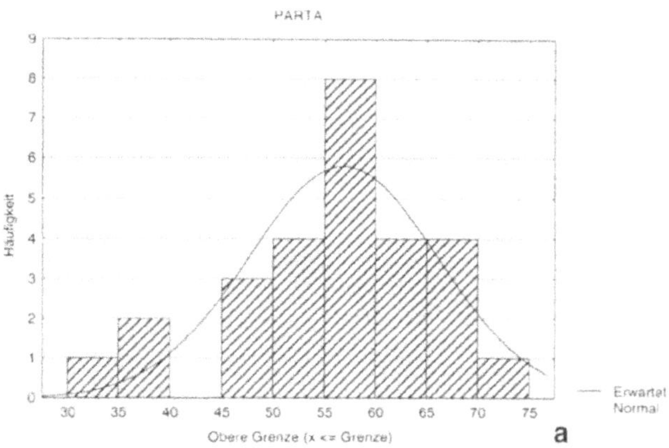

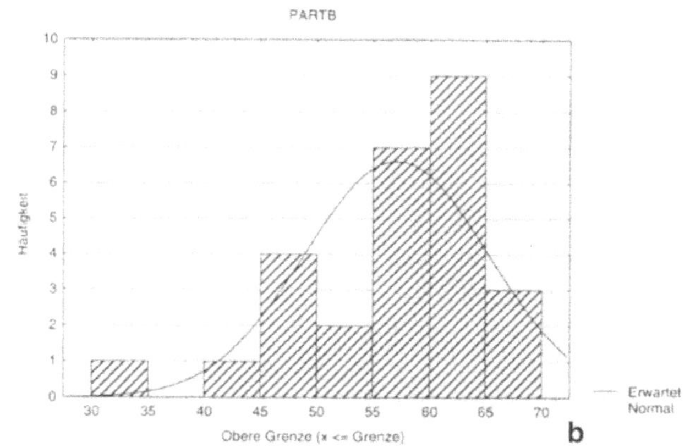

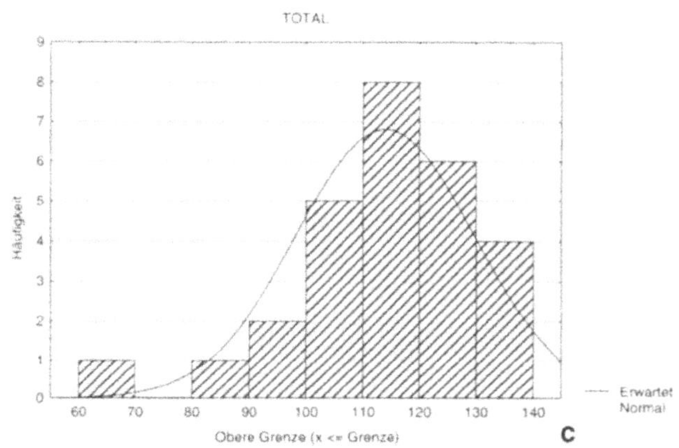

Fig. 1.

the final statistical evaluation. The 46 trainees had a total score of 2457 with a mean score of 53,41 reached by 59,35% of the trainees. Standard deviation from the mean score was 11.54. For part B one question was invalid and removed, mean score was lower (but also lesser number of questions) and was reached by 57.87% of the trainees. Thus there was no difference between the two parts of the exam. Out of 174 questions 6 (3%) were thus removed. For comparison at the ABNS exam of 1994, 23 out of 517 (4%) questions were removed before the final evaluation.

If, for instance, the mean score of part B had been significantly lower, e.g. reached by only 40% of the trainees, we would have evaluated the reasons for this and possibly found that some questions had been inadequately formulated, badly structured or too difficult to answer.

In the ABNS exam 147 out of 220 (67%) US citizens passed the MCQ. Foreign trainees who participate in the ABNS usually have much lower passing scores. As a control group last year, US medical students were tested with the same questions and they usually had a passing rate of 90%!!!

The passing score in our exam is decided upon each year after consultations in the Examination Committee. A fixed, yearly predetermined passing score of e.g. 67% is thus not used, nor do we use a control group. If we look upon a histogram of an exam, the distribution of trainees' results influences the decision (Fig. 1a).

Results of part A. (Number of valid questions were 90; only one candidate had between 70 and 75 correct answers, as seen at right of the abscissa).

Similarly, results of part B are shown in Fig. 1b. 84 valid questions, (3 candidates had between 65 and 70 correct answers).

Results of the whole exam are presented in Figure 1c.

Total number of questions was 174. Four candidates had between 130 and140 correct answers.

The Fig. also demonstrates that the one candidate with a very low score does not statistically influence the fit.

The scores are subjected to the normal Gaussian distribution to test whether distribution is statistically OK. From that we should decide the passing score. Each group of questions is scrutinized carefully.

In conclusion, we try to be fair to the candidates, use simple English words and have an external statistical expert to test the validity of our questions and results. From that evaluation a level for passing score of the exam is determined by the Examination Committee, usually with the mean score −2SD as the cut-off but always with a minimum of 60% correct answers as an absolute minimal requirement.

Secondary oral examination

The oral exam has never become the success we anticipated in the beginning, and in one year – 2001 – it had to be cancelled due to lack of participants. The first oral exam took place in Brussels in 1994 and exams are still carried out at that site. In the following it is important to notice that "EU-countries" and "European countries" are not synonymous. Potential candidates for our Oral Exam must have passed the primary MCQ exam, have a license to practice neurosurgery in *a European country*, must have had one year of practice in neurosurgery as an officially licensed neurosurgeon in *any European country*, and present a log book of operations performed independently after license has been granted. Initially they had to pay a fee of 1.200 DM, later 800 DM and presently 100 Euros [5]. The candidates are tested for 3 × 55 minutes on topics like brain and spinal diseases, peripheral nerves and other issues. Two examiners per session examine them consecutively. If insufficient performance becomes evident on some specific issues during the two first sessions, these topics are covered again in the last part of the exam by two new examiners. We use the American grading system (A, A−, B+, B, B−, C+, C, C−, D and E), "A" being an extraordinary result, "B" the standard, "C" not totally satisfactory and "D" definitely not acceptable for a professional function. If a candidate is given an "E", this candidate has failed the whole exam.

Having passed the oral exam, the candidate receives a **European Certificate** that has no "financial" or "accreditation" value as a license, but can be considered a true award. The best candidate of each year is awarded the "**Braakman Price of Excellence**", a book gift and a certificate.

The number of participants and pass/no pass are found in Table 4.

The total passing rate so far is 75.4%, thus being much higher than the passing rate of the multiple-choice exam.

Table 4. *Results of the oral examinations*

	Number candidates	Passed
1994	12	11
1995	7	6
1996	7	4
1997	6	6
1998	7	5
1999	7	5
2000	6	3
2001	0	0
2002	5	3

All details of the exams including the general rules are now published on the EANS Homepage *www.eans.org* [7]. Applications for exams and notification of results is now organized by the EANS Secretariat, in contrast to previously when the whole work was carried out by the members of the EANS Examination Committee.

Discussion

The problem we face is that the oral examination, in contrast to the written exam, costs money and does not give any legal rights to the candidate who passes, unlike the situation in the UK or in the US. The costs have recently been reduced significantly. Furthermore a candidate, already well integrated in professional life, may risk failing the exam and thus being personally and publicly humiliated [11]. Many potential candidates in the past have used these two reasons for not participating. Another important point is that most European countries today have a compulsory National Board Exam the trainees have to pass at the end of their training. The great disadvantage is that the EANS European oral exam – at least at present – is not equivalent to the National Board Exams and cannot "replace it" – so why take it?

One strategic goal of the EU is to provide a free exchange of persons and services, also within the medical services, as specified in the Directive 93/16 EEC of April 5, 1993. To meet these goals a harmonization of the training of medical specialists, in combination with quality assurance according to given standards will become mandatory. Considering the existing diversities among the countries of the EU in providing quality assurance for recognition as a specialist, a definition of standards with agreed levels of knowledge, practical skills and judgment is urgently needed. The

Table 5. *European Primary Examination September 1997*

Individual results in percent

Participant no.	Result of		Total
	Part A	Part B	
0001-3	62	59	121
0002-6	67	49	116
0003-9	76	64	140
0004-2	65	53	118
0005-5	67	50	117
0006-8	52	43	95
0007-1	61	53	114
0008-4	41	35	76
0009-7	44	42	86
0010-7	46	55	101
0011-0	54	50	104
0012-3	68	55	123
0013-6	63	51	114
0014-9	59	42	101
0015-2	64	58	122
0016-5	49	52	101
0017-8	56	44	100
0018-1	50	45	95
0019-4	64	53	117
0020-4	38	38	76
0021-7	48	38	86
0022-0	43	36	79
0023-3	64	56	120
0024-6	64	57	121

Table 6. *Results of trainee NN ("John Doe"), who failed the exam*

Result of John Doe	DID not PASS	35.1% correct answers
	Your result	Whole group
Total	35.1%	58.6%
Neuroanatomy	41.2%	63.3%
Neuropathophysiology	30.0%	58.0%
Neurology	14.3%	59.2%
General skills	50.0%	55.0%
Head injury	14.3%	49.7%
Brain tumours	48.3%	59.5%
Cerebrovascular disease	36.7%	55.7%
Peripheral nerves	50.0%	60.7%
Spine and cord	25.0%	56.5%
Neuroradiology	100.0%	87.7%
Paediatric and congenital	10.0%	61.5%

recent enlargement of the EU by additional 10 countries stresses the importance of such a demand. The European Examination must therefore become the accepted and agreed standard which can either be used by the national societies or used as a model when national societies or authorities prefer to organize this on a national level. A critical discussion of the actual European Examination therefore is needed to eventually secure the best possible solution.

Critical remarks to the present multiple choice question exam and the passing rate

As mentioned, the pass/fail score for the primary exam is determined by the Examination Committee, using statistical comparisons. Sixty percent of the correctly answered questions are the minimum number to pass (Table 5). For comparison, in the USA, 64% of correctly answered questions are needed and this percentage is remarkably consistent each year [4]. In the UK, the respective figure is between 64–69%. Despite the slightly higher pass score in the USA and the UK, a higher percentage of trainees pass the exam that means that they in general reach a higher average score as compared to the EU trainees. This may indicate that EU candidates are either less used to this type of exam, have more difficult questions, or have less comprehensive knowledge. This needs to be examined in more detail.

An important factor is the feedback if a resident fails the exam. In Table 6, the results of a candidate NN ("John Doe") are presented.

It is evident that this candidate had major problems in neurology, head injury and paediatrics (congenital disorders) and also remained below the average level of the whole group in most of the other fields. What can he learn from his results? Certainly that his efforts to acquire adequate theoretical ad hoc knowledge did not reach the anticipated levels.

In addition, the demonstration of his weakness in most of the main fields of our speciality may entice him to actively continue studying these topics specifically. He should recognize that his professional performance might be significantly hampered by lack of theoretical knowledge.

A feedback so far does not exist. In future a member of the examination committee or even better his local tutor, after revising the results of table 6, should discuss the results with this candidate and give him/her adequate support. It is therefore important to provide the Programme Director with the performance of his trainees in the individual test categories. Only this allows the Programme Director to take respective measures and adjust the curriculum, if needed.

Issues to be discussed in the future

Recognition or certification as a neurosurgeon should mark the successful completion of a well-structured training curriculum designed to train safe and competent clinical neurosurgeons [8]. The recognition or certification process is a very responsible decision and should be made as objectively as possible. The process itself and its quality have to be scrutinized from time to time! Is the present European examination – which is more or less a copy of the ABNS and the UK examination – adequate or can it be improved in certain aspects?

The written MCQ examination is designed as to test cognitive knowledge about topics related with neurosurgery. Questions include neuroanatomy, neurobiology, neuropathology, neurophysiology, neuroradiology, theoretical clinical skills, intensive care and all categories of clinical neurosurgery. The validity of the individual questions of the various subjects and of the entire examination can be tested and allows standardisation, so that each year's performance can be compared to the previous exams. In the written exam the assessment itself is as objective as possible. The real weakness is the selection of questions, whether they really represent the total amount of knowledge required for a neurosurgeon to make his surgical decisions as safe and correct as possible. How much ad hoc information is needed for instance in anatomy to perform operative procedures in the CNS or the peripheral nerves? How much of this anatomical knowledge must be immediately available in our memory? The question is easily answered for routine and standardised procedures like a lumbar disc or the removal of an acoustic neurinoma. For rare approaches is it appropriate to rely on memory or information systems, books, Internet can be used to update knowledge (clinically relevant knowledge). The MCQ can by no means tell neither the trainee nor the trainer whether the trainee will be a successful neurosurgeon.

The oral examination is thought to be a test of judgement and knowledge (how to use information) regarding the management of cases, including complications, outcome, etc. Typically case scenarios are presented and the candidates with appropriate scans, MRI s, etc. explain how they would manage the case and plan and perform an operation, if indicated. Complications and outcomes are discussed. By having 3 different sessions with 2 examiners each, examiner bias is reduced to a certain extent.

The oral exam in its present form cannot be considered an objective and standardised test because examiners often use personal case material of different difficulty, and this probably varies from examination to examination. Also individual examiners differ in their evaluation of the candidate's performance [8, 13].

Standard scenarios include subarachnoidal haemorrhage-, severe brain trauma-, brain tumours-, intensive care- etc.

In order to reduce this potential bias, more work needs to be done to validate (format) these case scenarios, weigh their difficulties and make the examiner's rating of the candidates' performance more objective. Even taking into account all these potential bias, the oral exam is still the best available technique to assess judgment and clinical performance.

The oral exam is presently offered 2 years after being recognised as a neurosurgeon. Experience so far has shown that this is not acceptable to the majority of candidates for different reasons, as discussed before. The Examination Committee therefore should consider to offer the oral exam at the end of training, which would make it part of a board examination and allow to accept both examinations as equivalent/supplement to a national examination within the EU.

Some additional instruments may be developed in the future to judge other relevant qualities of a candidate, such as operative skills on the one side and "social intelligence" on the other. The assessment of operative skills may be improved with the recent introduction of minimum and optimum figures for operative procedures required at the end of the 6-year training programme, and particularly by introducing competence levels for each procedure which have to be confirmed by the Programme Director (see "A structured Neurosurgical Training Plan"/K. W. Lindsay and "The new Neurosurgical Training Charter"/J. Steers, H. J. Reulen, K. W. Lindsay in this book).

This would give the Training Programme Director, who in fact is responsible for training the individual trainee, more responsibility when signing personally the level of competence acquired for each of the demanded operative procedures.

"Social intelligence" is a term comprising different qualities and personal characteristics, which are difficult to measure. Probably the best way is to review (study) the trainees' portfolio with his accomplishments and particularly the assessment forms for each training period signed by the trainers. In the USA, endorsement letters of practicing neurosurgeons in the community where the candidate works are required.

Conclusions

Efforts must be undertaken to convince national societies and authorities that in future a common European standard is mandatory for recognition (accreditation) of a neurosurgeon. The present European Examination can certainly be improved and become a model for such examinations.

Addendum 1. European examination in neurosurgery (Guidelines)

The European Examination in Neurosurgery consists of two parts:

The Primary Examination and the Oral Examination.

Both examinations may be taken on a voluntary basis and are prepared by an Examination Committee consisting of 12 program directors in Neurosurgery from various parts of Europe.

Primary examination

The **Primary examination** is a written, multiple-choice question examination (MCQ) consisting of 150–200 questions covering neurosurgery, neuroanatomy, neuropathophysiology, neuropathology, neurology, neuroradiology, fundamental clinical skills and other disciplines deemed suitable and important by the Committee.

These multiple choice questions have to be answered within 3–4 hours.

The Examination is prepared by the Examination Committee with the assistance of a professional institute for the design and analysis of examinations in medicine. This institute also carries out the analysis.

The examination can be taken once a year in August/September in two separate cities in Europe, either the same city where the annual European Course of Neurosurgery takes place or alternatively Uppsala, Sweden, provided there is a sufficient number of applicants.

The primary examination is open to all residents in accredited neurosurgical programs in Europe, and to all neurosurgeons with a license to practise neurosurgery in a European country.

It is advised that residents should not take the examination before their 4th or 5th year of training, otherwise the examination is generally considered to be too difficult. The level of the examination is intended to be comparable to the level of the Primary Examination of the American Board of Neurosurgery.

Participants agree that they are bound by the Committee's rulings regarding credentials and examination scores.

Candidates, fail or pass, may sit the examination as often as desired either for certification or self-assessment.

Fees are payable in advance and determined by the examination committee. They may vary at the discretion of the committee according to the costs of preparation and analysis.

The completed application form must be filed with the Examination Committee by middle of June.

The candidate must indicate on the form whether the examination is taken for credit toward certification or for self-assessment.

Oral examination

The Oral Examination is the second and final step of the European Examination. A pass at the oral examination is the only way to obtain the European Certificate in Neurosurgery.

Requirements to participate in this examination are:

- Evidence that the Primary European Examination in Neurosurgery has been passed.
- License to practise neurosurgery in any European country. A copy of this license must be submitted for inspection.
- At least one year of practice in neurosurgery as an officially licensed neurosurgeon in any European country.
- A logbook of operations performed independently during a consecutive period of 12 months after the license has been granted.
- Advance payment of the fee payable in Euro as specified on the application form. (approx 100 Euro).

The Examination Committee makes the final decision regarding a candidate's eligibility for the Oral Examination and potential certification after considering all available information pertaining to the entire process of certification.

The examination in the English language consists of three parts, each lasting one hour:

The first hour is dedicated to an oral examination by two examiners on operative neurosurgery of brain and skull.

In the second hour operative neurosurgery of spine, cord and peripheral nerves is covered.

In the third hour topics will be discussed that could not adequately be covered in the first two hours.

The examination is a clinical problem solving and patient management test. It is not a theoretical examination such as the Primary Examination. Case histories are given, and – where appropriate – X-rays, scans, MRI's and other visual aids are shown to augment the presentation and development of cases. Candidates explain verbally how they would proceed to evaluate or manage the cases and to plan and perform the proposed operations, if indicated. 3–6 cases will be discussed per hour.

Each of the three hours is conducted in an interview setting with two examiners, experienced neurosurgeons from a European country.

During these three hours the candidate will, therefore, meet six different European examiners, each of whom will give an independent score.

The final, combined score will be made available by mail within 14 days after the examination.

The best candidate will be awarded the Braakman Diploma of Excellence.

The candidates who pass this examination will receive **The European certificate in neurosurgery**.

This is a document that certifies that the owner has a good level of theoretical and practical knowledge in neurosurgery. It marks a successful completion of standard neurosurgical training.

It is not a license to practise neurosurgery in any European country. The European Certificate – at least at the moment – does not replace any national license. It is an award rather than a license.

If a candidate fails the examination once, a minimum of one year but not more than 3 years should elapse before taking the exam for the second time. A re-examination fee must be paid prior to the examination.

A candidate who has failed the Oral Examination twice must take and pass the Primary Examination again before reentering the certification process and retaking the Oral Examination. An additional year of practice data is also required. The candidate must again pay the examination fee.

Application forms for both examinations can be obtained from the EANS secretariat (stephanie.garfield@virgin.net; registration is possible via the internet *www.eans.org* – What's new – European Examination).

The responsibility for the European Examination rests with the Examination Committee of the EANS.

References

1. ACGM outcome project *www.acgme.org/oome/implement/rsvp.asp*
2. Adams JA (1987) Historical review and appraisal of research on the learning, retention, and Transfer of human motor skills Psychol Bull 101: 41–74
3. American Association of Neurological Surgeons (AANS): *www.neurosurgery.org/aans*
4. American Board of Neurological Surgery (ABNS): *www.abns.org*
5. Braakman R (1977) Experience with the EANS Examinations Acta Neurochir (Wien) [Suppl] 69: 88–92
6. Campbell CM, Parboosingh JT, Gondocz, ST, Babitskaya G, Lindsay E, De Guzman RC, Klain LM (1996) Study of physicians use of a software program to create portfolio of their self-directed learning. Acad Med (Wien) [Suppl] 10: 49–51
7. European Association of Neurological Societies (EANS): *www.eans.org*
8. Haff JT, Eisenberg HM (1997) Assessment of Training Progress and Examinations. Acta Neurochir (Wien) [Suppl] 69: 83–88
9. Kolmos A, Hjalmered JO (1993) Project-organized curricula in relation to basic and applied Science, long and short curricula and distance learning, in: SEFI Cahier nor 4: Project-Organized curricula in Engineering Education, Brussels
10. McDonald JM (1993) Mental readiness and its links to performance excellence in surgery. Kinetek, Ottawa, Canada
11. Palmer J (ed) (1996) Neurosurgery 96, manual of neurosurgery. Churchill, Livingstone, p 13
12. Physician Achievement Review *www.par-program.org/PAR-Inst.htm*
13. Picard J (1997) Experience with the United Kingdom Examinations in neurosurgery Acta Neurochir (Wien) [Suppl] 69: 93–97

Correspondence: Prof. Dr Jens Haase, Department of Health Science and Technology, Aalborg University, Frederik Bajers Verj 7 D-1, 9220 Aalborg Denmark. e-mail: jph@ist.auc.dk

Acta Neurochir (2004) [Suppl] 90: 115–119

Printed in Austria

XV Neurosurgical subspecialization: pros and cons

G. Schackert[1] and **H.-J. Reulen**[2]

[1] Neurosurgical Department, University Clinic TU Dresden, Dresden, Germany
[2] Neurosurgical Department, Ludwig Maximilians University, Munich, Germany

Introduction

In the past decades neurological surgery as a specialty has seen a burst of growth. As a result such multifaceted development has led to the fact that a single neurosurgeon might not be in a position to offer excellent expertise in all aspects of the speciality anymore. Consequently, groups of special interests have been forming in order to clinically and scientifically develop specific aspects of neurological surgery at a high level.

For these reasons, in Germany a committee for 'subspecialization' was formed, embedded in the constitution of the Neurosurgical Academy for Continuing Education (*Neurochirurgische Akademie für Aus-, Fort- und Weiterbildung* – NCAFW). The function of this committee is to critically examine the advantages and risks of developing such subspecialties and acquiring additional qualifications. In this review, we like to present the German concept which may serve as a basis for a broad discussion among the members of the neurosurgical community, not only in Germany but also in other European countries.

As a matter of fact, many departments have already adopted and developed special areas of interest within the specialty of neurosurgery. This movement cannot and must not be decelerated. However, it makes sense to reroute such developments in neurosurgery by means of clear definitions and timely planning. There is an urgent need to draft a general concept that would be feasible for all future subspecialties of neurosurgery, whereas the specific criteria and demands of training institutions and programs for the various subspecialties may be developed in an individual manner.

From postgraduate training to subspecialization (= additional qualification)

Chances and advantages

It seems that the only real possibility to practise and further develop our specialty at a high level of competence in all its breadth is to form special areas of interest and directed training of subspecialists. For instance, a neurosurgeon with an additional qualification in 'spinal neurosurgery' should be in a position to perform complex surgical procedures such as reconstruction of the vertebral body, tumor removal, stabilization etc., and at the same time should closely follow new developments, i.e. application of endoscopic procedures in spinal surgery, etc., in order to constantly widen his knowledge and hone his manual skills and techniques. He should also be in a position to represent his special area from both clinical and scientific aspects and to train younger colleagues of the department. On account of his high competence he should attract patient referrals which, otherwise, the department would not have gained.

Another prominent example is 'neurosurgical oncology' where various special techniques such as neuronavigation, intraoperative ultrasound, electrophysiological monitoring for determining eloquent brain areas (brain mapping), PET, functional MRI, stereotactic biopsy and many more come into play. Some of these techniques are frequently used and have become today's standards, while others are quite difficult and may be applied only to a small patient population. Presently there is a trend to acquire these techniques and to spend more time in treating patients requiring these techniques. If this development towards subspecialization is seen from a positive point of view, it broadens competence, knowledge and scopes of an improved training of specialists in a given department; moreover, such an aspiring attitude increases patient referrals and offers a considerable improvement of professional perspectives.

Risks and dangers

First of all, there exists the danger that the subspecialty will separate from the mother specialty, thus forming a subunit with demarcations of technology and personnel. Such a separation of subspecialties in the sense of complete independence should be avoided by all means. The neurosurgical service should remain one unit. All subspecialties should be part of the neurosurgical department and should not only take part in basic neurosurgical treatment (standard operations), emergency cases and training, but should also recognize these tasks as mandatory. The rights and obligations of a subspecialist should be clearly defined. The involvement of subspecialists in the emergency treatment also means that he keeps his skills in such treatment constantly honed.

It should be ensured that the right to perform a neurosurgical subspecialty procedure is not completely reserved to the acquirer of an additional qualification in that subspecialty. The non-acquirement of an additional qualification should not restrict or exclude performance of standard procedures, especially from the medico-legal point of view. The danger of undermining this principle in a legal trial is present; for example, in trying for compensation of loss, a lawyer may insist on the absence of an additional qualification of the neurosurgeon. Thus the concept of 'standard neurosurgical procedure' should be well defined. One of the decisive aspects in this matter is that training of a specialist in neurosurgery should include all theoretical and practical aspects in such a way that unrestricted practising of all of neurosurgery is permitted through board examination. A thoroughly trained neurosurgeon should be in a position to perform all standard procedures in neurosurgery. With the acquirement of a subspecialization, the surgeon should gain special depth of knowledge and expertise in that particular field of neurosurgery. Thus the task of neurosurgical subspecialization may be defined as the mastery of all conservative and operative standard treatment strategies, the treatment of complex and rare cases, and particularly the performance of highly specific, extraordinary procedures that demand advanced technological and technical dexterity in that area. It would be the task of the subspecialist to represent his area scientifically and develop novel treatment modalities. Successful new concepts offering a considerable improvement and, above all, simplification of an already existing treatment method should be included in the list of standard procedures, and thus be made available to all future neurosurgical trainees during their routine training.

Criteria for additional qualification in a subspecialty area of neurosurgery

In the following, the so-called "Institutional criteria", and the guidelines for training (Training Criteria) in a subspecialty area shall briefly be outlined.

Institutional criteria

For a neurosurgical department it is possible to establish a subspecialty area if the patient traffic within that area has reached a certain magnitude. The required minimum number of patients per year may be defined by a specifically entrusted work group and additionally be confirmed by the respective national neurosurgical societies. Alternatively, this may be organized on a European level. It may be concluded that large departments might tend to have more subspecialties while smaller departments may be limited to a few. For example, the implementation of 'spinal neurosurgery' may be possible in most of the clinics, whereas the necessary number of cases to establish 'pediatric neurosurgery' may be reached by only a small number of departments.

A department that aspires to establish a subspecialty should meet several prerequisites: a pre-defined minimal number of patients in that subspecialty area, related diagnostic departments and technology, interdisciplinary approach (for instance, neurooncology: tumor clinics, regular interdisciplinary meetings, library, access to neuropathology, neuroradiology, radiotherapy etc.). The institutional criteria for other subspecialties such as 'spinal neurosurgery' may look different. Thus, it would be the task of a subspecialist to organize and conduct the interdisciplinary approach according to such specified criteria.

Training criteria

Continuing education and training of a subspecialist demands the development of a training catalogue for that specific field in a similar manner as has been accomplished already in the United States. These catalogues are being developed by specifically charged work groups of a national society. At the European level, this would probably be a work group defined by the Section of Neurosurgery of the UEMS and/or the EANS. The guidelines for institutional criteria and the training catalogue for 'neurooncology', 'spinal neurosurgery', and 'neurosurgical pain management' that have already been published in the organ of the German Society of Neurosurgery *(Mitteilungsblatt)* are typical examples. Minimal duration of an additional qualification should be $1-1\frac{1}{2}$ years after board certification in general neurosurgery, judging from the experience of our colleagues from the USA.

The acquirement of an additional qualification in a neurosurgical subspeciality

When establishing a subspecialty for the first time in a department,

(a) the institution should fulfill the required criteria and
(b) the designated head of the subspecialty area should be able to fulfill the criteria of a subspecialty training catalogue.

When such a subspecialty meets all the institutional criteria and would be chaired by a qualified subspecialist, he may be formally nominated as a trainer for this subspecialty.

How can a specialist be trained to be a subspecialist in the future?

A candidate for subspecialization should have completed his training in neurological surgery. The subspecialization training should be offered only in such institutions where it does not compromise the training of residents in general neurosurgery. Training of residents should always have priority over subspecialization.

In Germany, it has been proposed to recognize a subspecialty qualification (a) by means of confirmation through the trainer and the chairman of the department, and (b) through the *Neurochirurgische Akademie für Aus-, Fort- und Weiterbildung* according to the criteria developed by the respective work groups and presidents of the German Society of Neurosurgery and the German Federation of Neurosurgery. A certification through the German Federal Chamber of Physicians (Deutsche Ärztekammer) or the State Chamber of Physicians has deliberately not been aimed at since adequate practical experience with the recognition criteria must be gathered primarily within the Neurosurgical Academy for Continuing Education. However, we plan to remain in close contact with the Federal Chamber of Physicians regarding these matters. If, at a later stage, the introduction of an additional qualification should be discussed in the Order of Postgraduate Training of the Federal Chamber of Physicians, then subspecialization in neurosurgery might fall under the category of a 'Qualification Upgrading Certificate'.

A list of possible subspecialty areas in neurosurgery

At the present point of time, training catalogues for the following subspecialties are being prepared:

- Neurosurgical oncology (completed)
- Spinal neurosurgery (completed)
- Stereotactic and functional neurosurgery
- Neurosurgical pain therapy (completed)
- Vascular neurosurgery
- Peripheral nerve surgery
- Pediatric neurosurgery.

Subspecialties should be large enough, it should be avoided that individually planned small areas of our specialty isolate themselves and form a 'subsubspecialty'.

Rights and obligations of a subspecialty

Furthermore, internal limitations of rights and obligations have to be described. It has already been mentioned that any tendency towards independence of the subspecialties from neurosurgery should be avoided. The chairman of a department carries final responsibility for the subspecialties practised in his department and has the right and obligation to organize the treatment of patients as well as the conduct of training residents including their rotational assignments. It may be specifically mentioned that the chairman or one of the staff members assigned by him is responsible as the Director of Training Program for student education and training of specialists as well as for the assignment of trainees to a respective subspecialty rotation. However, it is desirable to discuss and agree upon these matters with the respective subspecialist of the department.

The chairman of the department can delegate responsibilities for a subspecialty area to a staff member possessing an appropriate additional qualification. This subspecialist would be completely responsible for the treatment of patients in his area of interest; however, he still remains subordinated to the chairman. This means that diagnostic procedures, indications and operative therapy are administered according to the general guidelines of the department. The introduction of new treatment policies should be discussed prior to accomplishment (also in view of economical reasons). The subspecialist is obliged to train residents during their rotation in the respective area. Furthermore, those candidates showing interest in a subspecialization would be trained by the respective subspecialist. Subspecialization in a specific area also encompasses responsibility for research and development in that particular field. An academic subspecialist would be required to lecture and perform innovative research in his field of specialty.

Subspecialty: "Special Neurosurgical Oncology"[1]

The institutional criteria and the training catalogue of the subspecialty "Special Neurosurgical Oncology" may be presented as an example:

Minimum time for subspecialization amounts to $1\frac{1}{2}$ years. This may be undertaken after completion of neurosurgical training.

Subspecialization requires the following items:

1. Special knowledge, experience and skills in the indication and surgery of 50 supra- or infratentorial tumors and 20 spinal tumors in addition to the numbers required for general training in neurosurgery.
2. Knowledge of indication and surgery of at least 20 biopsies, with the aid of three-dimensional planning systems (e.g. stereotaxy, navigation systems) in addition to the procedures required for general training in neurosurgery.
3. Chemotherapy treatment according to established protocols in 30 patients, including follow-up examinations, awareness and treatment of chemotherapeutical side-effects (e.g. blood counts, prophylaxis of infections, antiemetics, disturbance of lung or kidney function etc.). Knowledge of handling chemotherapeutic drugs.
4. Knowledge and experience in radiosurgical procedures.
5. Participation in clinical scientific projects is recommended. Knowledge of good clinical practice (GCP) is especially demanded in clinical research.
6. Participation in at least two medical education meetings in neurooncology are required.

Institutional criteria for the subspecialty area "Special Neurosurgical Oncology". Medical centers or hospitals have to fulfill the following requirements:

1. Diagnostic institutions and techniques
   - Neuroradiology (incl. MRI)
   - Neuropathology
   - CSF cytology
   - Electrophysiology, incl. intraoperative monitoring
2. Treatment procedures
   - Surgery: routine surgery of supra- and infratentorial tumors and spinal tumors.
   - At least 60 gliomas, 30 meningiomas, and 30 other brain tumors annually, pediatric brain tumors, 25 spinal tumors/year (intra- and extradurally).
   - At least 30 biopsies with the aid of computer assisted three-dimensional planning systems (e.g. stereotaxy, navigational systems).
   - Radiotherapy, eventually in connection with radiosurgery.
   - Tumor outpatient clinic: regular follow-up of neuro-oncology patients.
   - Scientific research: Concomitant scientific research is desirable. Participation in multicenter studies, scientific-clinical work or basic science projects.
3. Neuro-oncological conferences on a regular basis:
   - The treatment of neurooncology patients should be discussed in regular interdisciplinary conferences with neuroradiologists, neurologists, neuropathologists, radio-oncologists and other disciplines that are involved in the tumor center.
4. Department library
   - A library with neuro-oncology literature and updated journals is required.

[1] These guidelines have been developed by a task force led by J.C. Tonn and G. Schackert

The subspecialty "Special Neurosurgical Oncology" can only be established in centers certified for neurosurgical training.

Conclusion

The need for subspecialization in neurological surgery is obvious. The increase in surgical and scientific knowledge, provided by the different subspecialties, will strengthen the field of neurosurgery. Its realization should be unanimously supported by the neurosurgical community.

References (for further reading)

Couldwell WT, Rovit RL (2002) Rethinking neurosurgical subspecialization. Surg Neurol 58(6): 359–363

Dwyer AP, Herkowitz HN, Benzel EC (2002) Controversies in spine: Should there be subspecialty certification in spine surgery? Spine 27(13): 1478–1483

Herkowitz HN, Benzel EC (2002) Controversies in spine: Subspecialty certification should not be a requirement for spine surgery. Spine 27(13): 1478–1483

Mainprize TG, Taylor MD, Rutka JT (2000) Perspectives in pediatric neurosurgery. Childs Nerv Syst 16(10–11): 809–820

[No authors]: Program requirements for residency/fellowship education in neuroendovascular surgery/interventional neuroradiology: special report on graduate medical education: a joint statement by the American Society of Interventional and Therapeutic Neuroradiology, Congress of Neurological Surgeons and American Association of Neurological Surgeons, American Society of Neuroradiology. Neurosurgery 48(2): 457–458

Ostertag C (1997) Subspecialty training in neurosurgery. Acta Neurochir (Wien) [Suppl] 69: 126–129

Piepgras DG (1997) Post residency subspecialty training in neurosurgery – The impact of subspecialty training on organized neurosurgery and resident training – benefits, responsibilities and liabilities. In "Training in Neurosurgery". In: Reulen HJ, Steiger HJ (eds) Acta Neurochir (Wien) [Suppl]

Correspondence: Prof. Dr. med. Gabriele Schackert, Klinik für Neurochirurgie, Universitätsklinikum Carl Gustav Carus der TU Dresden, Fetscherstr. 74, 01307 Dresden, Germany. e-mail: Gabriele.Schackert@uniklinikum-dresden.de

Important addresses

Address of Chairman JRAAC

Prof. Dr. T. Trojanowski
Department of Neurosurgery
University Medical School
Ul. Jaczewskiego 9
20-950 Lublin
Poland
e-mail: *Trojan@asklepios.am.lublin.pl*

Address of Secretary JRAAC

Prof. Dr. M. Zerah
Service de Neurochirurgie
Hôpital Enfant Malades
149, rue de Sèvres
F-75015 Paris
France
e-mail: *michel.zerah@nck.ap-hop-paris.fr*

Application Form for European Accreditation

to be downloaded from the internet:
www.eans.org
What's new: Accreditation of Training Centers

European Logbook

Electronic version can be downloaded from the internet
www.eans.org
What's new: Trainee Logbook
Also see: Information
Printed version is available from
Aesculap AG & Co. KG
P.O. Box 40
D-78501 Tuttlingen
Germany
Attn. Mrs. Eva Streit
e-mail: *eva.streit@aesculap.de*

European Charter on Training

to be downloaded from the internet
www.uems.be
Training/Formation – visitation – UEMS Charter on Visitation of Training

Evaluation Form

to be received from
Klinikum Großhadern
Neurosurgical Department
Co: Mrs. Ilona Anders
Marchioninistr. 15
81377 Munich
Germany
e-mail: *Ilona.Anders@med.uni-muenchen.de*

Author index

Index of keywords

SpringerMedicine

Alexander Baethmann, Jörg Eriskat,
Jens Lehmberg, Nikolaus Plesnila (eds.)

Mechanisms of Secondary Brain Damage from Trauma and Ischemia

Recent Advances of our Understanding

2004. VIII, 127 pages. Numerous figures.
Hardcover **EUR 98,–**
Reduced price for subscribers to "Acta Neurochirurgica": EUR 89,–
(Reduced price with approx. 10% discount)
(Recommended retail prices)
All prices are net-prices subject to local VAT.
ISBN 3-211-20932-8
Acta Neurochirurgica, Supplementum 89

Top level clinical and laboratory scientists present their most recent clinical and experimental findings and concepts. The well balanced contributions illustrate the enormous significance of the dialogue between both laboratory and clinic, ultimately for the benefit of the patients, and contribute to a better understanding of secondary brain damage from trauma and ischemia as basis to develop more effective treatment including drugs.

SpringerWienNewYork

P.O. Box 89, Sachsenplatz 4–6, 1201 Vienna, Austria, Fax +43.1.330 24 26, books@springer.at, **springer.at**
Haberstraße 7, 69126 Heidelberg, Germany, Fax +49.6221.345-4229, orders@springer.de, springeronline.com
P.O. Box 2485, Secaucus, NJ 07096-2485, USA, Fax +1.201.348-4505, orders@springer-ny.com, springeronline.com
Eastern Book Service, 3–13, Hongo 3-chome, Bunkyo-ku, Tokyo 113, Japan, Fax +81.3.38 18 08 64, orders@svt-ebs.co.jp
Prices are subject to change without notice. All errors and omissions excepted.

Springer and the Environment

www.ingramcontent.com/pod-product-compliance
Lightning Source LLC
Chambersburg PA
CBHW061219240926
51846CB00006B/1277
9783709172148